Sex & Back Pain

... restoring comfortable sex lost to back pain

By Lauren Andrew Hebert, PT

Second Edition

IMPACC Publishing, 89 Hillside Ave., Bangor, ME 04401

Published by:
IMPACC Publishing, 89 Hillside Avenue, Bangor, Maine 04401.
 (207) 941-0290; Fax (207) 941-8540;   (800) 762-7720

Printed in the United States by J.S. McCarthy Co.
Ist Printing, 1987.

Revised Edition of Sex and Back Pain;.....advice on restoring comfortable sex that has been lost to back pain.

Library of Congress Cataloging-in-Publication Data

Hebert, Lauren Andrew, 1952-
    Sex and Back Pain : Advice on Restoring Comfortable Sex Lost to Back Pain/
    Lauren Andrew Hebert.
    2nd Edition.
    p   cm
    1. Backache. 2. Sex. I. Title.
II. Title. : Advice on Restoring Comfortable Sex Lost to Back Pain.
ISBN 1-879864-00-2   LC 92-070997
                            CIP

617.564-dc20

Other books by Lauren Andrew Hebert, PT

Taking Care of Your Back

The Neck Arm Hand Book

Living with CTD

The Industrial Athlete

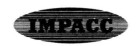

IMPACC Publishing, 89 Hillside Avenue, Bangor, ME 04401
(800) 762-7720

Acknowledgements

The production of this book has been a collaborative effort by several key people. Their sincere and sensitive input has contributed to help meet the objectives of this book. Thank you.

Artist:	David Whalen
Editor:	Adele Anderson
Layout:	Debbie McGee
Wordsmith:	Liz Hebert
Model:	Aaron Perreault
Professional Input:	Liz Hebert, LPN
	Patricia Creedon, PT
	Allen Wicken, PT
Production:	Bob Patterson
	Deane Jones
Printing:	J. S. McCarthy Co.

TABLE OF CONTENTS

Special Precautions!!

This book is written to teach people with back pain how to restore comfortable sex they may have lost due to that pain. Most back problems come from mechanical injury, aging or wear and tear to spine structures. These are the types of back problems we address in this book.

However: Back pain occasionally comes from serious diseases in internal organs. Pain from such diseases may be felt as lower back pain. There may or may not be other medical symptoms. Such people need to seek immediate evaluation by a medical doctor or osteopath.

This book can help you to restore sexual activities and rebuild a successful sex life that may be limited by your back problem. We will discuss pain control and strategies that can help restore spine strength and mobility. This book is not a substitute for proper medical evaluation and treatment. If you have a back problem you should consult a physical therapist, medical doctor, osteopath or chiropractor to develop your individual plan for back rehabilitation.

Back problems often lead to serious emotional, social or family problems. These can complicate your back disability and emotionally damage your entire family. A couple whose relationship is stressed by a disabling back problem should seek professional counselling to keep these complications from destroying the family. This book is not designed to be a replacement for such counselling.

Our recommended sex techniques are based on evaluation of methods likely to be most successful for people with back problems. Over 200,000 copies of a clinic version of this book have been distributed to back pain patients since 1986. It is important to remember, however, that there is no advice guaranteed safe or effective. Each case is unique. What works for one person may not work for another.

When you are attempting sexual activities keep in mind that you need to proceed with care and caution at all times. Go slowly and respect the limitations of your body. Nothing in this endeavor is guaranteed safe or effective. Your objective should always be to take good care of yourself. Enjoy your recovery!

Lauren A. Hebert, PT

All is Not Lost!

Life with back pain can be a nightmare.
The losses, the changes, the fear
can be worse than the pain itself.
But...you can recover! All is not lost.

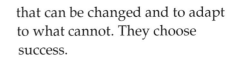

Back pain problems are very common, eventually striking eight out of ten people. Back problems are the leading cause of disability in the United States, costing nearly $80 billion annually in health care and lost production. The effects go far beyond pain and financial costs. It can destroy lives and families. But all is not lost. Most people do recover from their back problem. Even those with permanent disabilities continue with their lives and achieve great success. These people face their problems head-on, to change the things that can be changed and to adapt to what cannot. They choose success.

You already know that pain is only part of the stress with which you must live each day with your back problem. Back pain causes you to suffer many losses. You can lose many important aspects of your life to pain and disability. You may lose comfort, independence, security and happiness. You live with pain and disability every day of your life. You may suffer loss of employment, financial security, recreation and self-esteem.

Some of the toughest changes you may face is in your relationships with the people around you, particularly within your family. Family members no longer see you in the same light. Your roles have changed for them and they view their relationship with you as changed. Each of you may resent these changes. The pain and losses all create emotional stresses such as depression, anger and constant worry. This can make your back problem worse.

Pain can affect your nervous system in ways that may make you more sensitive to many emotions. The constant stimulation of pain centers in the brain can make you more depressed or angry. These changes also can make you more sensitive to pain. It becomes a self-perpetuating circle that can make your problems progressively worse.

Back pain can easily come between partners, no matter how strong their relationship. The stresses caused by back problems can be both emotional and physical. Back pain can cause loss of a satisfying sexual relationship with your partner. Sex may now cause pain. Fear of pain can further cripple sexual enjoyment. The effects of pain on your sex life can result in many bad feelings such as fear, anger, guilt and frustration. The pleasure of sex may be replaced by conflict and frustration. Your relationship with your partner can suffer severely. This makes your other problems much worse.

Your comfort, your peace of mind, your happiness, your job, your role in the family can all be damaged. You feel cheated out of life and your self-esteem may be seriously diminished. Loss of self-esteem, loss of sexual ability and loss of loving communication all feed the fires of misery for you and your partner. The cycle becomes self-destructive and seemingly hopeless...**if you allow that to happen!**

Back pain can create many cycles of personal suffering and destruction. Be aware that your back pain need not control your life. You can decide to take control. You can decide that back pain will not destroy your life or your family. All is not lost!

Restoring relations with your partner can be a big step toward reversing many of these stresses. These destructive cycles must be broken and replaced with rebuilding a healthy relationship. This, in turn, can significantly reduce your pain problem. You and your partner must learn to share feelings more closely and be willing to explore various sex techniques. This book is a guide for **both** of you to break free from the vicious cycle of pain, frustration and failure caused by painful sex. By reading this book you are already moving toward the goal of rebuilding your relationship, your family harmony and your life.

Anger and Guilt

*Feelings of anger, guilt and blame
are a typical part of back pain.
But now it is time to let that go and move on.*

Back pain is invisible. No one except yourself truly knows what it is like. Some people around you may not fully accept your pain because they cannot see it. There is no obvious evidence of your pain. There is no scar or bleeding for others to see that proves your complaint is real. Some people may question your honesty. You begin to suspect that no one believes you. You live with feelings of suspicion and betrayal, particularly with your family and spouse. This is very stressful and adds to your pain and suffering.

You live every minute of every day around your pain. It becomes your focus in life. It may be all you talk about, or you may even refuse to mention it. Either way, your pain becomes the focus for your family. This brings you guilt while creating worry and resentment within

your loved ones. You all fear the uncertainty of the future. There may be anger at what your pain has brought to the family. Everyone worries that the situation will last forever or become worse. This situation can become very stressful to everyone.

Anger may become a big part of your life in this situation. You may close out your spouse and other family members. They may, in turn, close you out. You end up playing destructive "games" of manipulation and punishment. You and your partner must recognize what back pain can do to you as a couple and take steps to fix it.

You also may feel betrayed by your body. We all believe we are indestructible, until we get hurt. Then we feel betrayed by our body and by life in general. You no longer feel strong and ageless after a back injury. Your life changes. Your roles in your family change. You cannot help resenting those changes and your family may resent them as well. You may feel you have brought stress to your family. You may fear that your family views you with anger and betrayal, which only increases your resentment and guilt. The damage to everyone's happiness can be extensive...if you allow the situation to continue.

Recovering a fulfilling sex life depends upon you and your partner understanding the difficult feelings that often result from pain, frustration and anger. You must both understand how these feelings get in the way of your sexual relations. Sex is no longer fun and erotic. Instead, it becomes burdened with conflict and expectations of failure. Sex no longer communicates positive feelings and sharing between you. You should be sharing intimacy, not anger. To be successful you must break that cycle. You have a responsibility to yourself and your loved ones to overcome these problems.

Successful recovery of good, healthy sex requires that you discover sex techniques that are as comfortable as possible for your back. But before that can happen, you must rebuild positive attitudes about sex with your partner. You need to understand that anger, guilt and fear are typical complications for both of you in this situation. Discussing these issues to get past the destructive feelings is vital to your recovery. Once you begin to communicate, not only about your pain but also about your feelings you can then discuss how you and your partner can rebuild healthy loving sex.

Sexuality versus Sensuality

*It is not your physical performance that counts;
it is your attitude.
It is the sensuality that we enjoy sharing.*

Sex is a physical act that requires physical performance. Your spine must be able to move and to hold positions during sexual intercourse. A back problem can seriously limit your physical capabilities. You may lack strength, mobility, flexibility, endurance and comfort. Fear of pain and failure can further limit your abilities and your patience.

Back pain, by limiting your physical abilities, can limit your sexuality as well. Back pain does not, however, limit your sensuality. Sensuality is the romance and excitement of sex. This is the source of the pleasure of sex. Sensuality supports a loving sexual relationship better than sexuality. Sensuality is your **attitude** toward sex with your partner. Restoring sex lost to back pain requires you to place an emphasis on first restoring your sensuality.

You are more likely to fail during sex if you focus only on your physical performance. Enjoyment of the experience of sharing can be lost to your critical judgement of your performance and its results. You end up judging yourself and your partner rather than appreciating the sharing of feelings and enjoyment. This takes away from sensuality and reduces the role of healthy sexual love in a relationship.

It is vital that you keep in mind that you are **not** the only one having a problem with sex. Your partner is also living with the problem.

Open communication is the key to restoring good sexual relations. The basic strategy for restoring sex begins with open discussion and deliberate planning by both of you to restore a close and sensual friendship.

Start by agreeing that you will now commit a special effort to your relationship. You must both let go of at least some of the ill feelings that may have developed around this problem. Accept that anger and frustration are typical of this situation. Realize that many of these ill feelings are actually directed toward the problem, not the person. Successful recovery of your sexual and sensual relationship will require some understanding of the pain issues. Decide to let go of the anger and move forward.

This book is a starting point and a structure for recovery. Go through the book together. Plan a "date" or series of "dates" devoted to gently rebuilding a sensual relationship around your back problem. Let this book lead to some sensual ideas that you may try together. These things have to be planned at this stage to avoid failure. Plan an evening or afternoon alone together. Let that planning create some erotic excitement for both of you. Plan the romance. Plan how you will avoid pain and frustration. Agree upon a strategy and how you both will deal with pain.

You may wish to avoid the times and places where failure and conflict have become a habit. An afternoon encounter may help you avoid the fatigue and discomfort you often feel at the end of a long day. Sex after a long and difficult day is often doomed to failure. Planning your date to occur in a setting other than in the bedroom, such as a private "picnic" in the living room or elsewhere, can help break a cycle of repeated failure in the bedroom.

Each person has a unique idea of romance and is aroused by different things. Take the time to think about what might be stimulating for both yourself and your partner and share some of your ideas with each other. Decide to explore areas that you both find exciting but non-threatening.

There are numerous ways of creating a sensual atmosphere that are popular with many people. Candle light dinners, soft music, dancing, lingerie, perfume or romantic movies are just a few examples. Sharing a bath or shower or a gentle massage can help to relax you and create a sensual mood.

For some people, recreating a situation from the past that holds special romantic meaning for you both may be a welcome experience. A favorite restaurant, a special song, certain articles of clothing or a particular location where you remember having felt especially loving or romantic. The kind of atmosphere recreated from pleasant memories can be both stimulating and relaxing.

Think about an atmosphere that will create a sensuous mood for both of you and plan to make it happen. The extra effort you put into creating the right atmosphere can make all the difference. Make preparations and allow anticipation to create sexual excitement, but without demands or unreasonable expectations that could lead to failure. Let the anticipation be seductive. Plan not to fail in your lovemaking. Agree that encounters with pain during sex will not lead to anger or guilt or

blame, even if pain brings things to a halt. Accept that some ill feelings may occur, but be prepared to let them pass. Plan how you will avoid excessive physical demands on your back before sex and during sex. Decide ahead of time how you will enjoy each other with minimal demands and stress.

Your objective is to enjoy sharing sensuality, touch and intimacy. Agree ahead of time that you will not push physical demands too far. Agree also that any encounters with pain will be allowed to come and go without anger, guilt or feelings of failure. Pain is to be expected and allowed to pass without conflict. In a later chapter we will discuss pain control strategies that you can fit into your lovemaking. Sharing, communicating and enjoying each other is the goal. Explore gentle touching and erotic play that you may have, perhaps, forgotten or neglected in your relationship.

You should accept that sexual desire may be, for now, somewhat reduced by pain and fear of pain. Do not impose unreasonable expectations on yourself or your partner. Accept that it can be very sensual and sharing simply to lie close together, especially if no demands are being made on anyone's part. Non-sexual touching and holding one another, talking and listening are all part of sensuality and sexuality. Make this a new courtship experience. You have not given up on sex, you are rebuilding it.

We will discuss various strategies for pain control, communications, relaxation, and physical approaches to successful sex. It is important that both of you examine these chapters to plan for success!

Touch

Touch may be the most basic and meaningful form of communication that can exist between two loving people. The way that we touch each other can express a wealth of feelings without the use of words.

Gentleness and a deliberately slow pace are the keys to sensual touching. Always begin in a non-threatening manner that is not overtly sexual. There are many ways to touch your partner that will both relax and stimulate. Gently touching your partner's face or hair can be very sensuous and an excellent way to communicate warmth and caring. By taking

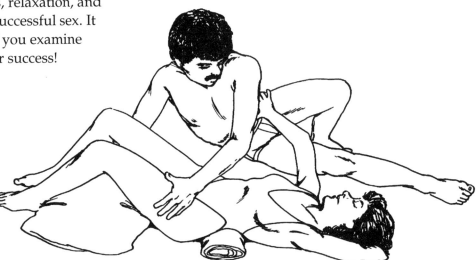

your time and being as gentle as possible you will show your patience, understanding and desire to do whatever is necessary to make the encounter a success.

A period of gentle, non-sexual touching will help you and your partner to relax and feel comfortable with physical contact. Fear of pain can create physical and mental anxiety. By taking the time to create a sensual, yet non-threatening atmosphere through gentle touching, you can alleviate some of the anxiety that often creates more pain.

There are many highly sensitive and responsive areas of our bodies that many people never take the time to explore. Take this opportunity to discover as much as you can about your partner and what he or she finds pleasurable. Even if one or both of you are uncomfortable with verbally communicating your needs or desires, by slowly exploring your partner's body and being sensitive to his or her reactions you may find yourself learning a great deal more than you ever imagined you would.

Be patient with yourself and your partner. Let your instincts about the needs of both of you be your guide. Remember that your sensual encounters need not always lead to actual intercourse to be successful. If the cycle of pain and anxiety is to be broken, it must be done with patience and gentleness.

Too Shy to Discuss Sex?

Don't let this destroy your relationship.
Speak up. Discuss the situation. Decide to succeed.
It is worth it to dare to talk about it!

Many people are just too shy to talk about sex, even with their sex partner. It is good to respect the privacy and deeply personal nature of sex but not at the expense of communication. Many people let themselves and their partner suffer frustration and lack of satisfaction because their sexual and sensual needs are not being met. They may feel cheated in life because they cannot bring themselves to discuss sex. They may also feel guilty and angry with their partner and with themselves because needs and desires are going unsatisfied. This can be a tragedy, particularly when all they really need to do is talk and listen to each other. Open and honest communication is a major part of love. Love does not let you read someone's mind.

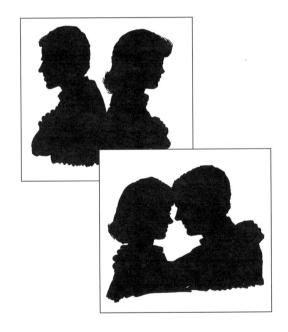

If you or your partner have difficulty with such a discussion, try underlining a few important sentences in this book and giving it to your partner to read. Perhaps pencil in "What do you think?" in the margin next to some important paragraphs, inviting a response. Exchange comments in this way several times.

A back problem can cause a lot of stress. The loss of your sex life makes the problem much worse for both of you. This book can help guide you to recovery. But you have to discuss sex to get it back! If you avoid talking about sexual needs because you are too shy, you may ultimately find yourself facing a disaster that need not have happened. Your relationship is worth the effort to overcome your shyness and discuss these matters openly with your partner. Consider what you have to lose and what you have to gain. It is worth it, isn't it? Dare to speak up and express your needs without demands, threats or blame.

You can rebuild your sex life by first rebuilding your closeness, communication and sensuality. This requires gentle understanding of your needs and those of your partner. This book will provide specific advice on sex techniques that help protect your back. These are physical techniques. You must provide the emotional caring that allows them to succeed.

How Your Spine Works

*You must understand how
your spine works to understand and
control your back problem.*

Anatomy: The Working Parts

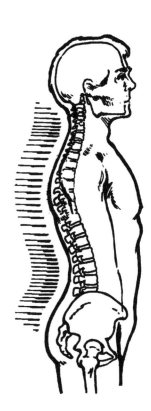

Your spine is a complicated and very sensitive machine with many moving parts. These parts are under very heavy and constant weight-bearing loads. Your spine has two basic jobs: Maintain a **stable**, upright posture and be **mobile** to provide movement. Your spine is strong, hard-working and sensitive. It must hold your body (and whatever load you may be carrying) upright and balanced over your two feet. At the same time, your spine must be able to move these loads efficiently in any direction.

Your spine is under constant movement, weight-bearing and position stress whether you are lying down, sitting, standing or walking. It is a challenging job for the spine to be both **mobile** and **stable.** This is a very difficult demand and makes the spine vulnerable to injury. That is why you must use your back properly, and why your spine must be kept strong and flexible.

Spine Parts:

Your spine is made up of some important working parts:

1. The bones of the spine are called **vertebrae**.

2. The vertebrae are separated by cushions called **discs**.

3. The vertebrae pivot on their **joints.**

4. The spine is held together by **ligaments.**

5. The spine is moved by **muscles.**

6. This is all monitored by very sensitive **nerves.**

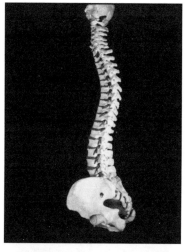

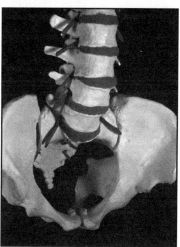

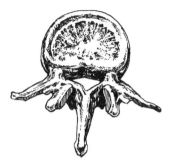

Vertebrae

The bones of your spine are called **vertebrae.** These are small blocks of bone stacked one on top of another. There is a hole running down through these bones for your spinal cord. This stack of vertebrae is called the **spinal column.**

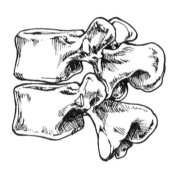

The spinal column is curved to work like a spring. These curves allow the spinal column to handle heavy loads efficiently. The neck curves inward; the middle back curves outward; the lower back curves inward. This lower back is called the **lumbar region** of the spine. The lumbar region curves inward, forming a mild "swayback" curve. This curve is called the **lumbar lordosis.** In this lordosis curve position the joints, discs, muscles and ligaments are in their strongest and most stable position to protect your back. This lordosis curve gives your lower back its strength and mobility for work.

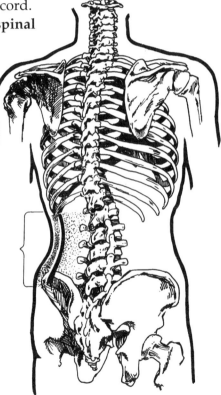

Discs

Each **vertebra** is separated by a cushion called the **disc.** The disc is a ring of very tough fibers surrounding a soft jelly center. The ring is called the **annulus.** The jelly center is called the **nucleus.**

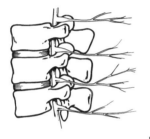

The nucleus acts like a small fluid ball between the vertebrae. The vertebrae roll or pivot over this nucleus as the spine bends and moves. The disc cushions lifting loads and the shock of walking. The disc is vulnerable to injury because of the heavy loads and forceful movements pushing and pulling across it.

It is important to know what happens to your discs when you bend your spine. Bending forward causes the vertebrae to tip forward over the nucleus. This stretches the back of the annulus. The pressure on the front of the disc pushes the nucleus back against the back of the annulus, stretching it further. This back wall of the disc is weak and can be damaged by too much of this stretching. This is how discs often rupture. The stretching action can rip open the back wall and the nucleus may be pushed through it.

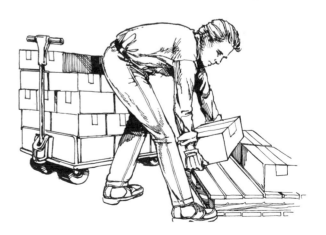

19

Bending your spine backward does just the opposite. The vertebrae tip back over the nucleus, stretching the front of the disc. This causes the nucleus to push forward toward the front of

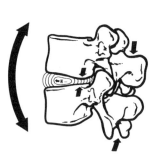

the disc. But this is not as damaging to the disc because the front wall of the disc is much stronger than the back wall. Mild backward bending of the spine often provides relief to the over-worked back wall of the disc that is stressed by bending and lifting loads all day.

Facet Joints

The discs separate and cushion the front portions of the vertebrae. The back parts of the vertebrae, however, are connected to each other at their joints. Each vertebra overlaps the one below it, much like roof shingles overlap each other. This overlap is called the **facet joint.** Each facet joint acts as a hinge, a pivot point of movement between the vertebrae. These joints are extremely sensitive. They are filled with very sensitive nerve endings that monitor movement and position. This helps us maintain balance and posture. These nerve endings are also very sensitive to stress, strain and pain.

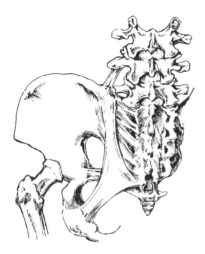

Ligaments

Ligaments hold the spine together. Ligaments are very tough bands of connective tissue that bind together the vertebrae and their joints. This is to limit movement and hold the spine together. These ligaments run along all sides of the spine to provide support in all directions. They enclose the vertebrae, discs and joints to make the spine stable. It should be noted that the ligaments surround the discs to prevent rupture except on the back side of the disc where the ligament is weak and thin, even missing on some people. This is another reason that the back wall of the disc is often ruptured.

Muscles

The **muscles** of the spine are very powerful. They do two jobs at the same time. They must hold you in an upright posture all day long. They must, at the same time, move and work the spine. These muscles are very strong. They

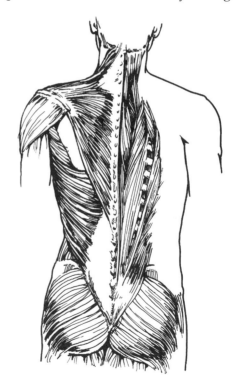

21

are also very sensitive, filled with nerve endings that sense movement and position and pain.

These muscles not only move and posture the spine, they also protect the other spine structures during loading and bending. Good muscle strength and flexibility are important to protect joints, discs, ligaments (and the muscles themselves) from being torn apart by bending or lifting loads.

Nerves

The spine is a strong, stable, mobile, delicate and sensitive machine. This requires a rich

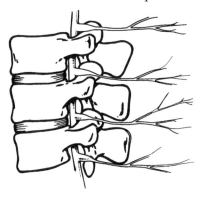

supply of very sensitive **nerves.** These nerves monitor movement and position to tell the muscles how to maintain balance and coordination. They also feel the pain of injury or disease. These nerves are scattered throughout the ligaments, joints, muscles and other structures of the spine.

The nerves come from the **spinal cord,** which runs down through the vertebrae. The nerves branch off the spinal cord from between the vertebrae. These branches, known as **nerve roots,** pass between the disc and facet joint. This can be a site of irritation between discs, facet joints and nerve roots.

Blood Supply

These structures in the spine require a **blood supply.** The blood supply provides the nutrition these tissues need to survive and to repair daily wear and tear. Poor circulation to these tissues causes them to break down.

Movement is vital to good circulation of spine tissues. This movement pushes blood and other fluids throughout the spine tissues. This allows weight-bearing tissues like the discs and facet joints to "sponge up" fluids that provide nutrition. A spine that has stiff joints, damaged discs or tight muscles may not get the nutrition it needs due to lack of movement. This can increase damage and slow repair.

Back Problems

*Knowing how problems begin and how they are treated
can give you more understanding and control
over your back problem.*

Muscle Spasm

Muscle spasm is an uncontrolled locked muscle contraction; a cramp. This spasm shuts off circulation to the muscle and causes a build-up of irritating acid waste products. The lack of circulation and build up of acid wastes irritate the muscle, producing pain and more muscle spasm. This reduces circulation still further, creating a cycle of pain causing spasm causing more pain causing more spasm. This impairs spine movement. The lack of movement also reduces circulation to discs, joints and ligaments.

Muscle spasm is often not the only problem. Spasm is usually caused by another irritation. Nearly any back problem will produce muscle spasms. Injury to the bones, joints, discs,

ligaments or the muscles themselves will all produce muscle spasm in response to the pain. Even diseases not related to the spine, such as

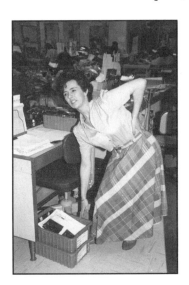

kidney stones or reproductive problems, can produce muscle spasms. Emotional stress and chemical imbalances in the body also can contribute to muscle spasm.

Muscle Strain

Muscles can be strained or torn. A forceful pull on the muscle may cause it to rip. This causes bleeding, irritation, pain and spasm. This rip may be the result of a heavy load placed on the muscle or by a forceful contraction effort by the muscle. A rip can occur if the muscle is weak, lacks flexibility or is working in an over-stretched position.

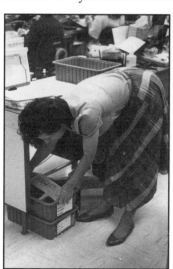

Slipped Disc

Discs do not "slip." The proper term for this is "bulging disc," "ruptured disc" or "herniated disc." The ring of the disc (annulus) can weaken with age, excessive work loads or abuse by its owner. This allows the nucleus of the disc to push and bulge the back wall of the annulus during bending, causing the annulus to "balloon" out. This is a bulging disc. The bulge may come and go over a period of time.

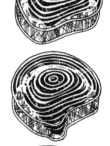

If the annulus ring of the disc finally breaks, the nucleus may be pushed out. This is a ruptured disc or herniated disc. The nucleus of the disc has been pushed through the annulus ring. It may then press against ligaments, joints, blood vessels and nerves. This can produce severe pain, numbness and paralysis in the back and legs.

Discs also can shrink with age. This is called a degenerated disc. As the disc thins, the space between the vertebrae is reduced. This shifts more weight-bearing load onto the facet joints leading to stiffness, arthritis or other joint problems.

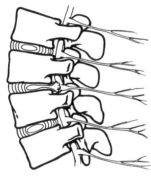

Ligament Sprain

Bending the spine too far, especially with a load, can place too much pull on the ligaments. These ligaments may rip, especially if they are not being adequately supported with strong back muscles. This injury can be extremely painful.

A torn ligament can leave part of the spine unstable, leading to further injury. On the other hand, the ligament may heal with scar tissue, making part of the spine excessively stiff. This scar tissue is easily torn again to produce another injury.

Facet Joint Sprain

The facet joints can be injured if they are jammed forcefully together or if they are pulled too far apart, ripping their ligaments. This can cause severe pain in these very sensitive joints. The injury may lead to internal scars that stiffen the joint. This stiffening can then lead to further damage to the joint over time.

A sprain or over-use can cause a joint to swell much like a sprained ankle. This swelling causes pressure in the joint, irritating nerve endings that can lead to pain and muscle spasm that stiffens the joint. The problem gets progressively worse.

Bending the spine forward forcefully may tear the ligaments holding the joint together. This can leave a joint unstable and easily injured again. Joints can be jammed together when the spine is forced backward or twisted. This may occur suddenly with a forceful sprain. More commonly, sprains occur gradually by prolonged or repeated reaching or twisting. This occurs particularly in people who stand all day or who are repeatedly lifting above their shoulders. Sprains also can be caused by repeatedly twisting the body, as in moving loads from one direction to another.

Years of use, abuse and injuries eventually wear out the joint surfaces making the joint stiff, reducing motion and encouraging more injury. This is degenerative arthritis. This arthritis can make the joints grow larger, pushing against nearby spinal nerves, creating a condition called spinal stenosis.

Sacro-Iliac Sprain

The base of the spine sits in the pelvis at the sacro-iliac joint. This is where the lower back and hips come together, making a very stable joint that is usually difficult to sprain. Certain conditions, however, can make this joint unstable. Disc problems can weaken the ligaments that support this joint. Foot and leg problems also can place abnormal stress on this joint. Certain female hormone changes such as pregnancy also can weaken the ligaments that support this joint.

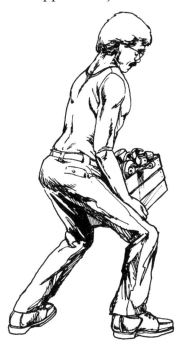

Referred Pain

Back pain may have nothing to do with a back problem! Diseases in organs deep in the body may be felt in the back, producing back pain and muscle spasms. This "referred" pain must be considered when back pain is felt with no obvious physical injury. The source of referred pain may be a sign of a tumor, a kidney problem, infection or female disorders.

Referred pain may be suspected when there is no specific injury, when you can find no position of comfort, when pain comes on gradually or when the pain cannot be reproduced with certain test movements. This requires immediate medical attention to identify the source of the pain.

Pain

Damage to spine tissues mechanically strains nerve endings in the injured structures. The damaged tissues release chemicals that can further irritate nerve endings. This mechanical and chemical irritation of nerve endings produces pain.

Pain is a very strange sensation. Once it gets started, it can be very difficult to stop. Once the pain finally goes away, it can easily return with only a minor irritation. The longer you have a pain, the more sensitive you can become to pain.

There is a pain "cycle." Injuries stimulate the pain nerves. The pain nerves tell the muscles to tighten to "splint" or lock up the injured area. The muscles can suffer spasms when they "splint". This reduces circulation to the muscles and causes a build-up of acids in the muscles. This can produce more pain and splinting and spasm.

Stiffening of the injured parts reduces movement in the joints and discs. Joints need movement to remain healthy. Lack of movement reduces circulation and allows rapid deterioration. The discs need movement. Movement allows the discs to "sponge" fluid in and out of the disc. Lack of movement greatly reduces the feeding of the disc. The disc can no longer support itself or repair its damage in this situation.

Pain also affects the brain. Constant daily pain can change brain sensitivity in ways that can lead to depression and other emotional problems. This also can cause the brain to become more sensitive to pain. Personal emotional problems can quickly become severe. Family problems, anger, frustration, alcohol and drug abuse all make these problems much worse. This is a very common and serious complication to back pain and must be treated along with the injury. The physical and emotional effects of pain can make the original injury become a long-term disabling problem that is very difficult to manage.

Understanding Pain

It is often difficult for both the pain sufferer and his or her partner to understand some of the effects of living with constant back pain. It may seem at times that the pain sufferer has had a complete personality change with periods of intense depression and anger. A person with a great deal of unmanageable pain may appear frustrated and intolerant with no patience for family members or friends. This kind of behavioral response to pain can be confusing and stressful for all parties involved. Often, the pain sufferer is as confused and dismayed by these behavioral changes as those around him/her.

Pain and disability can frequently cause a response of anger, resentment, fear, frustration, inadequacy, helplessness and even hostility in the sufferer. These kinds of negative feelings can become as disabling as the injury itself if they are not confronted by all concerned. By ignoring the emotional and psychological aspects of pain you may be helping to create a "domino" effect that can become highly destructive. Do not allow pain to put a wedge between yourself and those who care for you. Do not allow frustration to destroy the patience and tolerance you need to help a loved one in pain.

If you feel that you need help dealing with some of these issues, don't be afraid to speak with your physician or therapist. They can help you to confront both the physical and emotional effects of your pain. By helping you to understand your pain and your response to it, they also will be helping you to deal with it. Try to focus on your recovery rather than your injury. Channeling your frustration in a positive direction can be very helpful in shortening the recovery process. Allow your loved ones to help you. Don't push them away because you are feeling helpless or inadequate. Let them be a part of your recovery and share in your success. They are feeling just as frustrated as you are.

The family members of a person who is suffering from back pain need to remember that their loved one is often at the mercy of the pain that he or she is experiencing. Be patient with mood changes and sudden fits of depression or anger. If your loved one does not appear to be the same person since the onset of pain, remember, the "old person" was not in that pain. It may appear that the pain sufferer is angry and striking out at you, but what he or she is really angry at is the pain itself. Try not to take these feelings personally. Keep in mind that what you are experiencing is just another effect of that person's pain. Continue to care and be patient and respect the sufferer's need for solitude or venting of frustration. As much as you wish you could, you cannot take the pain away. Instead, do what you can to help your loved one through the difficult moments.

Causes of Back Injury

Back injuries come from wear-and-tear, work demands, work habits, accidents and poor self-care. Most back problems are caused by the habits of the victim. Most of us create our own back problems. It is how we choose to use and care for our back that leads us to our misery.

Bending: Your spine is designed to be held upright. But we spend most of our time bent forward. We bend forward to sit, work, play, even sleep. The more time you spend bent forward, the greater the daily wear damage to your spine. Think about it! How many hours per day do you spend bent forward?

Bending the spine forward often stretches the low back muscles to the point where they lose too much strength to protect the spine from injury. The ligaments are also placed on a weakened stretch during forward bending. The facet joints are in an unstable position. The back wall of the disc (annulus) is placed on a weakened stretch while the nucleus is pushed backward against it, risking bulge or rupture. How far you bend, how often you bend and how much time you spend in this position will determine the amount of wear damage.

Twisting: Repeated twisting can damage the spine. Twisting can over-stretch certain ligaments and muscles, weakening them. Twisting also pinches facet joint surfaces together. Twisting also can damage the annulus ring of the disc. Damage builds up gradually until, one day, a seemingly minor task causes major pain and injury.

We normally lose twisting mobility as we get older. Our spine tissues gradually stiffen. Stressing these tissues with repeated twisting work can lead to an injury as the aging process progresses. But this can be prevented and even reversed if you can restore good flexibility!

Poor Flexibility: Poor flexibility is a leading cause of back injury! Tight muscles limit your movement. A stiff body works much harder to do a day's work. Lack of flexibility allows far greater damage to occur during bending and twisting. Discs, joints and ligaments require normal movement for adequate circulation. Reduced movement can reduce feeding and repair of these tissues. A stiff body works harder and cannot adequately recover from injury.

Tight hip muscles and hamstrings are especially bad for the spine. These muscles can stiffen hip movements that are important to help the spine work efficiently. Reduced flexibility of these muscles will increase work loads on the spine and can lead to spine injury. Tight jeans do the same thing by limiting hip mobility!

Poor Posture: Posture is how you hold your spine during the day. Your posture is determined by your habits and your flexibility. Normal posture has a slight inward arch (lordosis curve) in your lower back. This curved posture allows you to use proper mechanics and gives nutrition to spinal tissues. It is the best position to tolerate "loading" to the spine (lifting, pushing, pulling, carrying).

A "flat" low back lacks a lordosis curve. It is straight. A flat low back bends the spine slightly forward from its normal curved position. A flat lower back compresses the discs, reducing their nutrition. Muscles and ligaments may be slightly over-stretched, weakening them.

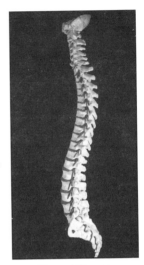

Normal Curves

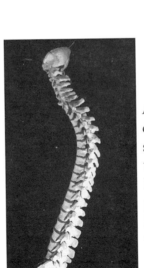

Flat Low Back

A flat low back is often caused by too much sitting, prolonged forward bending and tight hamstrings. Repeated or prolonged forward bending allows the spine to stiffen toward this forward-bent position. Tight hamstrings (the muscles in the backs of your thighs) pull down on your pelvis (the bone you sit on), which pulls the lower back lordosis arch into a flattened position.

Too much lordosis curve is called "sway-back". Sway-back places the lumbar part of the spine in a constant backward-bending posture. This can cause excessive compression of the facet joints and tight muscles. Sway-back may lead to excessive fatigue and discomfort at the end of the work day due to pressure on the facet joints and tight muscles.

Sway-back is caused by weak belly muscles, tight back muscles and tight hip muscles. Sway-back is often the result of prolonged standing, particularly on a cement floor. It also can be caused by excessive work with the arms reaching overhead. Pregnancy and obesity also can cause sway-back.

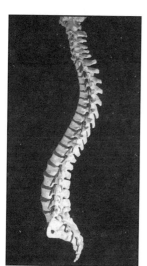

Sway Back

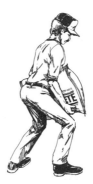

Poor Job Design: Some jobs can be designed to reduce the physical stress needed to perform the work task. This is known as "ergonomics". Poor job design, however, may require excessive bending, reaching, lifting or stressful postures. Examples of poor job design include:

- moving a load that is too heavy
- moving a load too often
- moving a load too far
- twisting with a load
- work that is too high, too low or too far to reach
- bad chairs, cold temperature, vibration, noise and clutter in the way

Your Personal Work Habits: Do you make your job more difficult than it needs to be? Do you arrange your work in ways that require bad positions or movements? Do you choose

33

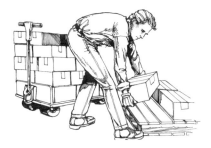

to use improper lifting habits? Do you take chances with your back? Many people let themselves get hurt.

This is the only back you have. It earns you and your family a living. It allows you to enjoy comfort. Your back must last a lifetime. It can do that only if you choose not to damage it with bad work habits. Your responsibility is to:

1. Arrange your work tasks in ways that reduce reaching, twisting, bending and excessive lifting

2. Use proper lifting and posture habits

3. Take proper care of your working back by doing frequent, on-the-job stretching and after-work exercises.

Poor Physical Fitness: Cardio-vascular physical fitness is your body's ability to deliver oxygen from your lungs to your bloodstream to your working muscles. Muscles need oxygen to support life. Physical fitness is good heart, lungs and circulation to deliver oxygen to the working muscles. Poor fitness reduces oxygen delivery to the muscles. This causes working muscles to run out of fuel, leading to weakness. The result can be an injury. People who are not in good general physical condition have more back injuries than healthy people.

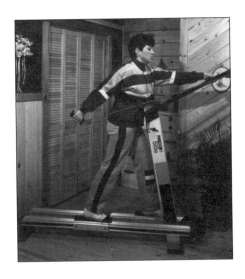

Your back needs proper care to keep it working for a lifetime. Keeping fit is the key! A daily walk, bicycling, cross-country skiing, aerobic exercise classes can be great for your body and your life. A treadmill, stationary bike or ski machine at home can be a great investment.

Smoking: Smoking can add damage to your back. Nicotine from tobacco gets into your blood and can damage connective tissue. Tobacco use also reduces circulation and oxygen in the blood. This can weaken protective muscle strength and reduce repair of daily wear.

Nutrition: Your body needs protein and certain vitamins to repair worn musculoskeletal tissues. A balanced diet provides the raw materials your body needs for repair. Poor nutrition leads to less repair of worn tissues. Eating disorders, poor eating habits and dangerous diets can add to your injury risks. A balanced diet provides what your body needs for work and repair.

Overweight: Have you ever carried a twenty pound bag of groceries all the way across the grocery store parking lot? Have you ever held a small child in your arms for a prolonged period? Did you notice how quickly you became tired? Try carrying around that weight all day. Just a few pounds of extra body weight can create a lot of extra work for your spine. This leads to excessive fatigue and extra wear on your body. Exercise that reduces weight will help your back.

Stress: Stress on the job, at home or anywhere can set you up for a back problem and can prevent back pain from getting better. Stress can stiffen and weaken protective back muscles and increase pain sensitivity.

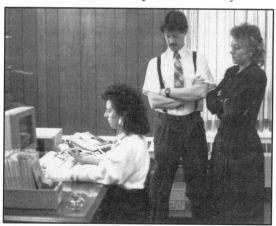

Back Treatment and Recovery

You can control pain, restore function and prevent reinjury.

Treatment for Back Problems

Treatment of back problems has three stages: control pain, restore function and prevent reinjury. Most people seek help for the first stage (control pain) and ignore the other two. This leads to a back problem that does not go away. Back pain is caused by mechanical back problems. The mechanical problems must be fixed before the pain will go away for good. Treatment must go beyond pain control to include restoration of strength, flexibility and safe back work skills. The following is a list of treatment strategies for managing back problems:

Rest: The best immediate care of a back injury is to go to bed and let the back injury heal itself. Injury and inflammation need early rest to repair themselves. But bed-rest must be limited to only a few days. Too much bed-rest can create more back problems. Two or three days of bed-rest can be very effective but it can quickly produce severe weakness, stiffness and poor circulation to back structures. Muscles rapidly become weak and lose flexibility. Joints get stiff and become over-sensitive. Discs become starved of oxygen and nutrients. These changes can prevent recovery. This may then lead to more bed-rest as the patient experiences reinjury due to ongoing stiffness and weakness. Brief bed-rest can help a lot but prolonged bed-rest can cause problems.

Prolonged bed-rest and inactivity also can produce emotional problems that complicate recovery and make life miserable. Emotional problems are very common with daily pain, lack of activity and absence from work. These make the physical problems worse! You and your family can suffer great stress.

Treatment by bed-rest should include a rapid return to walking, exercise and other activities within a very few days. Bed-rest should be limited to days, not weeks. Strength and mobility must quickly be restored.

Medications: Medications can reduce pain, inflammation and muscle spasm. They can speed recovery and help you tolerate return to activities. Like bed-rest, medications reduce symptoms only. They do not restore spine function. A quick return to activity and exercise is necessary to restore back strength and flexibility.

Medications can be dangerous. Ask your physician or pharmacist for complete instructions. Immediately question them about medication problems or side-effects. Always avoid over-use of medication.

Physical Modalities: Heat, ice, ultrasound and electrical stimulation can improve circula-tion and reduce pain. These modalities are provided by physical therapists to reduce symptoms but they do not restore spine function. Modalities are used to help you tolerate return to activity and your back exercises.

These modalities stimulate nerves that can turn off pain, open blood vessels and relax muscle tension. This can be important to preparing your back for sexual activity and recovering your comfort after sex.

Massage: Massage can be very healthy for muscles and connective tissue. It can reduce spasm and improve circulation. However, massage does not restore strength. It can be quite effective for some people with chronic muscle pain problems. But, again, it is exercise that will restore long-term muscle function and comfort.

Sharing massage can not only reduce pain and create relaxation, it also can be a form of communication and closeness to lead you into sexual activity. This can be a very important part of a couple's sharing of sensuality and sexuality.

Manipulation: Manipulation is when a doctor or therapist moves the joints of the spine with their hands. This may be a very gentle procedure (mobilization) or a more intense, sudden force (thrust manipulation). Manipulation should be performed only by chiropractors, osteopaths, specially-trained medical doctors and physical therapists. The purpose of manipulation is to stimulate the nerves of the joints in ways that can reduce pain, spasm and restore mobility. Manipulation is usually accompanied by exercises that build strength and flexibility.

Surgery: Surgery does not fix a bad back. Surgery may help some people with certain severe back problems but it can do even more damage. Surgery usually tries to remove ruptured disc material that may be pressing on nerves. Surgery should be limited to those people for whom nothing else has adequately helped. It may offer the only hope for certain seriously ruptured discs. It should be viewed as an option of last resort. A few people with serious nerve problems (such as a loss of bowel and bladder control) require surgery

immediately to avoid permanent nerve damage.

One of the most important parts of surgery is the rehabilitation after the operation. Surgery requires extensive physical therapy following the procedure to bring maximum recovery and minimum risk of reinjury. This therapy takes the form of pain control, exercise and education.

Physical Therapy Physical therapy is a physical, mechanical and educational approach to correcting the causes of the back problems. A physical therapist is a specially-trained medical professional who uses a combination of treatment strategies that include:

a. physical modalities to control pain and inflammation

b. massage to reduce muscle spasm and restore tissue mobility

c. exercises to build flexibility, and strength

d. education to make the patient a motivated expert on their back problem, to stay in shape and avoid reinjury

In the early stages immediately after an injury the physical therapist will try to control pain with the physical modalities. The therapist will quickly add various exercises to restore strength and flexibility.

Exercise: Exercise is key to recovery. Movement must be started as soon as pain and inflammation will allow some activity. Movement, strength and flexibility are necessary to restore circulation, healing and back function.

Exercises start with very gentle movements. They quickly progress to more demanding stretching and strengthening. Exercises restore joint mobility, muscle flexibility, strength, circulation and endurance. Certain exercises also may help damaged discs improve their circulation and reduce bulging. People with a back problem should have exercises specifically designed for them by their physical therapist or doctor. Different patients often need different exercises. We will describe a set of exercises designed to keep a back healthy, strong and flexible. These are designed to prevent an injury. Please refer to that chapter later in this book.

Education: This is the most effective back treatment available! The patient must become an expert on their back problem and normal back mechanics. They must be trained and motivated to use and care for their back properly at all times. Becoming an expert on your back gives you the best chance of recovery from a back problem or avoiding a back problem. That is the purpose of this book.

Back Recovery Exercises

Long-term pain control comes only from restoring the physical function of your spine. This includes muscle strength, muscle flexibility, joint mobility, and endurance. These functions can be restored only through specific exercises. Such exercises must be properly designed and the back sufferer must be motivated to perform them as instructed. This process is best designed by a professional physical therapist specializing in back care. The physical therapist is the most qualified expert on exercise therapy for back pain.

Flexibility is vital to the working spine, particularly during sex. You must be able to assume positions comfortably, move freely within those positions, and comfortably move out of the positions with minimal strain. You need adequate strength to stabilize and protect your spine during sex, plus enough endurance to make it through the activity without discomfort.

Exercises start with gentle movement and stretches, progressing to more vigorous strengthening as the back pain patient recovers ease of movement. The following illustrations demonstrate a typical progression of exercises for back function recovery. Patients are instructed to perform these gently, always keeping their efforts within the limits of pain. You should not perform any back exercises that cause pain. Some mild stretching discomfort is O.K. during some procedures, but pain that persists after exercise is a signal that the exercise is not appropriate or the effort is too much.

Standing Back-Bend Stretch:

Stand with your feet apart, hands on your lower back. Lean back gently. Hold 3 seconds. Repeat 3 times. You also may find this helps you avoid pain by doing this stretch after any sitting or bending activities (or after sex).

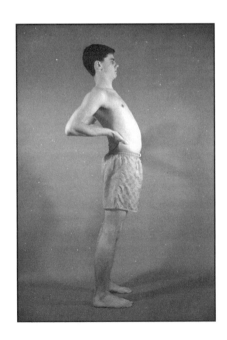

Prone on Elbows:

Lie on your belly. Prop your upper body up on your forearms so that the lower back sags inward. Relax 15 seconds in this position. Lie flat, then repeat 3 times.

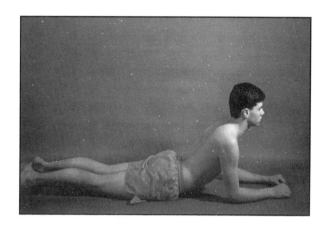

Prone Press-up:

This is a more advanced stretch. Lie on your belly. Place your hands under your shoulders. Press up your upper body so that the lower back sags inward. Hold 3 seconds. Repeat 3 times. Be gentle! Avoid this if it hurts.

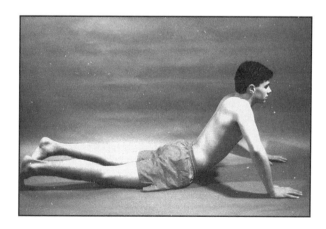

Hamstring Stretch:

Lie on your back. Bend one leg up and grasp your thigh. Hold your thigh straight up as you stretch your leg straight at the knee. Hold stretch gently for 20 to 30 seconds each leg. This will be somewhat uncomfortable.

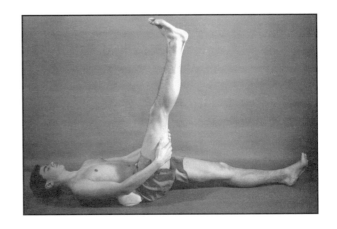

Hip Stretch:

Lie on your back. Hold one knee to your chest, keeping your other leg flat. Stretch 30 seconds each leg.

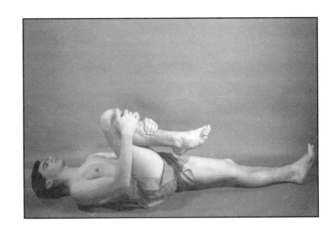

Lumbar Stretch:

Lie on your back. Bring your knees to your chest and hold them in with your hands. Stretch gently 30 seconds.

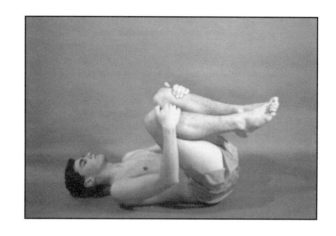

Middle Back Mobility:

Get on your hands and knees. Arch your back up like an angry cat for 3 seconds, then let your back sag like an old horse for 3 seconds. Keep elbows straight. Move up and down gently 5 times.

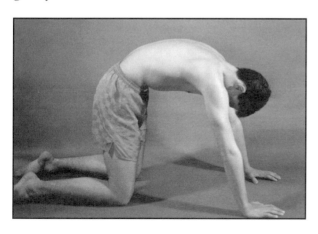

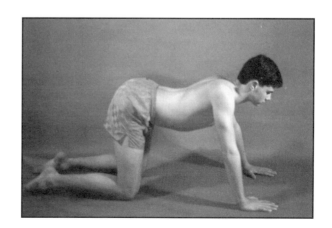

Middle Back Torsion:

On your hands and knees, reach under your body with one hand. Reach under and toward your opposite back shoulder. Hold twist stretch gently for 3 seconds. Stretch each way 5 times.

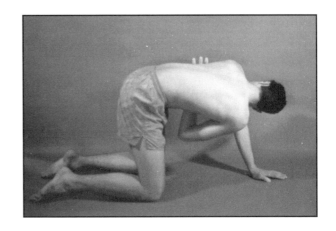

Joint Stretch:

Lie on your side with your legs bent up toward your chest and your chest curled forward toward your legs. Rotate your chest back so that the chest faces up. Stretch 20 seconds. Repeat with other side. Avoid if painful.

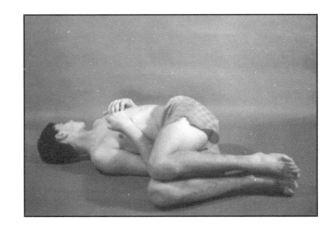

Obliques Strengthening:

Lie on your back with your legs bent. Cross your arms over your chest. Roll onto one shoulder and sit up sideways just a few inches. Hold 2 seconds. Relax, lie back, and roll to the other shoulder. Sit up sideways just a few inches. Hold 2 seconds. Repeat to fatigue.

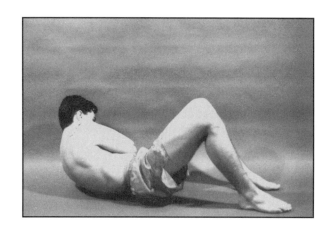

Hip Bridging:

Lie on your back with your legs bent and your feet flat. Raise your buttocks 6 - 8 inches. Hold 3 seconds. Relax. Repeat 10 times.

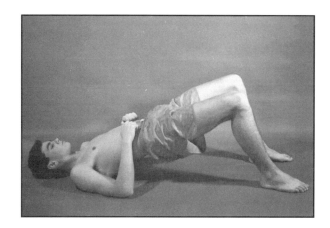

Hip Power Bridge:

Lie on your back with your legs bent and your feet flat. Raise your buttocks 6 - 8 inches. While holding your buttocks raised, lift and straighten one leg. Hold 3 seconds, then replace that leg and straighten the other leg as you continue to hold your buttocks up. Repeat 3 - 5 times.

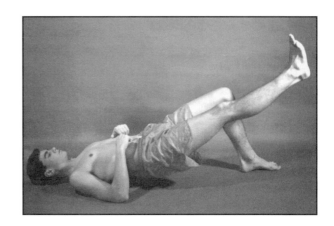

Upper Back Strength:

On your hands and knees, raise and reach forward with one arm. Hold 3 seconds. Switch to reach forward with the other arm. Repeat 5 - 10 times.

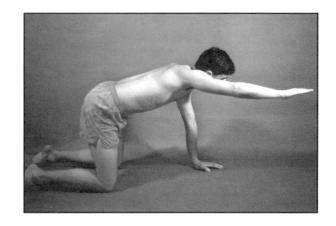

Lower Back Strength:

On your hands and knees, raise and reach back with one leg. Hold 3 seconds. Switch to reach back with the other leg. Repeat 5 - 10 times.

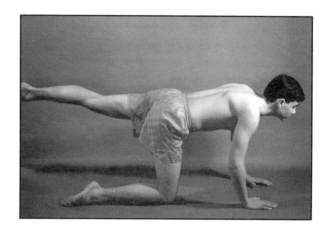

Full Back Strength:

Combine the two previous exercises. On your hands and knees, reach out with the opposite arm and leg. Hold 3 seconds, then switch. Repeat 5 - 10 times.

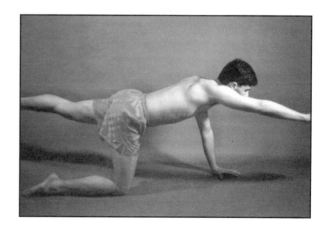

The very best overall exercise for back pain is walking. As in all exercising, it must be kept within the limits of pain. Walking produces rhythmic movements of the spine in its proper patterns of motion. This increases circulation, mobility, strength and endurance of all the structures of the spine working together.

If it is not possible for you to walk outside because of bad weather or difficult terrain, you can check and see if you have a health club or YMCA with an indoor track near you. Even your local mall can be a good place to walk in bad weather. You also might consider purchasing a cross-country ski machine, treadmill, stationary bike or stair-step machine. Avoid rowing machines.

Avoiding Reinjury

One of the most common problems of back pain is recurrence. Just when you think that your problem is going away, it hits you again. The key component in avoiding reinjury is to commit to using your back properly always and forever.

Lifting: First, don't lift unless you have to. If you must lift, keep lifting loads light and small. Second, do it right. Spread your feet, tuck your chin, arch your back slightly and squat. Lift with your chin tucked, your back upright and slightly arched and your knees bent.

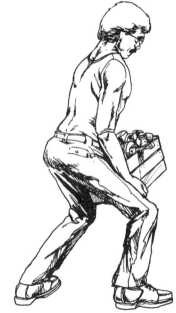

Bending: First, squat; don't bend. If you must bend or lift, frequently stretch into a gentle back-bending stretch. Keep all movement slow, gentle and within the limits of comfort.

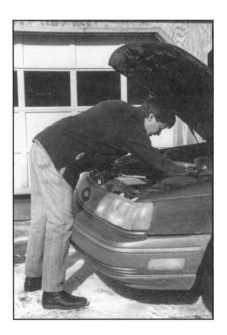

Don't become over-confident when pain is under control. When pain limits you don't get angry and respond by abusing your back. The reinjury is often more severe than the original injury. You must commit to using and caring for your back properly forever. It is the only one you have!

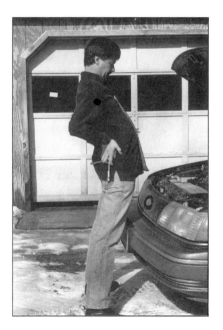

Pain Control

Develop your personal pain control strategy
that will enable you to enjoy sex in comfort.

Your physical abilities are limited by your pain sensitivity as well as by your back's stability, strength and stamina. Your capacity to tolerate sex greatly depends on all of these. Reducing pain and restoring back functions are the objectives of back rehabilitation programs and a pre-requisite to full recovery of your sex life.

Pain sensitivity can be reduced through pain medications, relaxation training, exercise and physical modalities (heat, ice, electrical stimulation). These pain control strategies attempt to reduce the sensitivity of the nervous system as it responds to the stress of physical activity. Each of these is effective for certain situations. You need to identify one or more procedures that can effectively control your pain. Using these procedures before, during and after sex

can greatly improve your tolerance of the physical demands of lovemaking.

Non-medication physical modalities such as heat, ice or electrical stimulation offer the pain sufferer safe and effective self-treatment for pain. The objective of self-treatment is to identify what works best to control pain encountered during daily activities. Most people rely on heat. Dry heat provided by a heating pad or heat lamp is usually not as effective as moist heat provided by a moist heating pad or hot shower. Heat should be limited to no more than twenty minutes, with aggressive precautions to avoid burns.

Applying ice has been shown to have surprising pain control effectiveness for many people, often more effective than heat. Although using ice may not be comfortable initially, it becomes very comforting after two or three applications. Ice is a top choice for pain control by many physical therapists, even for people normally bothered by cold weather. Ice therapy affects the body quite differently than a cold environment. Ice may be applied with gel cold packs available from most drug stores or through ice massage.

Ice massage calls for rubbing an ice cube directly over the painful area for five minutes. One convenient technique is to place a popsicle stick or spoon in a paper cup of water. Store a few of these in the freezer. Simply peel away the cup from the ice for treatment. The stick or spoon will provide a handle for comfortable application of ice massage. This will feel very cold, then hot, then numb. Not comfortable, but usually very effective!

Many chronic back pain sufferers use a small device that delivers mild electrical stimulation through skin pads placed around painful body parts. This is known as T.E.N.S. (transcutaneous electrical nerve stimulation). The T.E.N.S. device is prescribed by a physician or physical therapist and requires training in its use by the patient. Effectiveness varies from useless to miraculous among sufferers. One key to successful use of T.E.N.S. is proper set-up, electrical frequencies and patient training in proper use.

Relaxation

Another pain control strategy is relaxation training. Physical activity presents the risk of pain. Activity may lead to anticipation of pain. This creates tension, and tension can easily lead to pain and muscle spasm. The anticipation of pain can be as crippling as pain itself. This damaging tension-pain cycle can be easily corrected with **relaxation exercises.** Relaxation exercises can be performed just before sexual relations, following sexual activity and even during sex.

Relaxation Exercise

Lie on your back in a quiet setting. Place one or two pillows under your legs.

Extend your toes and feet backward as you inhale for three seconds. Relax your feet as you exhale for five seconds. Repeat three times gently. (You need not tighten any of these muscles very hard for the relaxation response to be effective.)

Next, tighten your thighs as you inhale for three seconds. Relax your thighs and exhale for five seconds. Repeat three times gently.

Then tighten your buttocks as you inhale for three seconds. Relax and exhale for five seconds. Repeat three times. (Skip any part of this that hurts.)

Tighten your belly and inhale for three seconds. Relax and exhale for five seconds. Repeat three times.

Clench your fists, shrug your shoulders and inhale for three seconds. Relax and exhale for five seconds. Repeat three times.

Tighten your face as you inhale for three seconds. (Do not clench your teeth!) Relax and exhale for five seconds. Repeat three times.

Then quietly tell yourself you are very relaxed at your feet, your legs, your back, your arms and your face. Consciously feel the relaxation.

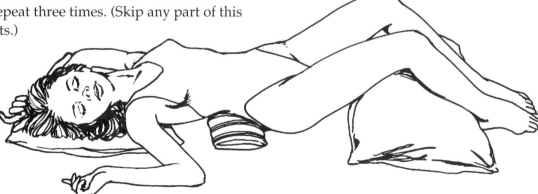

One of the best resting positions to relax a tired, sore back is the 90/90 position. Simply lie on your back on a firm surface such as the floor. Place your legs on a chair or ottoman so that your knees and hips are both bent and resting in a 90 degree right angle. This is usually one of the most relaxed and least stressed positions you can provide for your back.

You will need to develop some form of convenient and effective pain control to help you succeed in your recovery of sex. This not only offers help in controlling pain, it also provides you with greater confidence and less fear of pain during sex. Heat, ice massage or relaxation exercises can be applied before sex to build your tolerance to physical activity. These may be repeated after sex to reverse any pain you may have encountered. You can even incorporate a pain-control break into your sexual encounter if your back problem is particularly brittle and sensitive.

Pain medications are often important and effective treatment for back pain sufferers. You must be cautious, however, not to let pain medication block out your back's response to excessive physical demand or strain. These medications are designed to reduce inflammation, relax spasm and control pain. Do not let medications "mask" or hide damage. Medications require strict supervision of an M.D. or D.O. physician. You should closely follow the instructions of your physician and pharmacist. You should seriously question any unusual responses to medication and be very careful with narcotic-related drugs.

Sex Techniques for the Brittle Back

Even a serious back problem need not halt sexual activity. You can create sexual enjoyment and pleasure around your back problem.

Sex Techniques For the Very Brittle Back

For many people a back problem gets in the way of sexual activity. You may be in too much pain to tolerate any sex at all. But you have to start sometime, somehow. Each of you may be feeling some anger, guilt and fear. Your attempts at sex may have caused pain that adds to the anger, guilt and fear. You must break that cycle...together.

The actual lovemaking techniques we will discuss here are for those with a painfully fragile back problem, one that physically tolerates very little. Actual genital intercourse may be impossible for some people with a very brittle back problem. These people need,

at first, to use other sex techniques that do not put their back at risk.

The person with a very brittle back should begin by concentrating on the sensual romantic strategy described earlier. Once you are together in this environment and sharing the mood, you can proceed in a very relaxed and leisurely manner. The person with the brittle back should take a passive role in love-making at this stage. It is vital that you avoid frustration and impatience with each other as well as with yourself. Giving stimulation can be as erotic as receiving it. Seek to please both your partner and yourself. Share.

Plan to bring your pain under control before starting. Use whatever pain control techniques you have identified as effective. Apply heat, ice, massage or relaxation exercises, perhaps even incorporating them into your communication and foreplay. Share this as part of your mutual touching and relaxation. You may need to repeat your pain control techniques during and after sexual activity to keep pain under control, trying to keep sex as pain-free as possible. Try not to accomplish too much at one encounter. Plan to frequently shift position slightly to avoid discomfort. Rest frequently as needed. Plan this as part of an agreed-upon strategy.

You may or may not tolerate stimulation to orgasm at this time. If that is all you can handle for now, accept it. You will get together again. Recovery can be a slow process and at this stage success is not measured by achieving orgasm. Sharing touch and sensuality is the goal for now. Do not judge the quality of your sexual experience by orgasms, especially early in your recovery.

The partner with the back problem should be positioned so that the lower back is supported and relaxed. Lie on the back on a firm surface with the legs placed on one or two pillows. Some find it comfortable to have a small hand towel rolled or folded and placed under the lower back to support a slight arch (Figure 1).

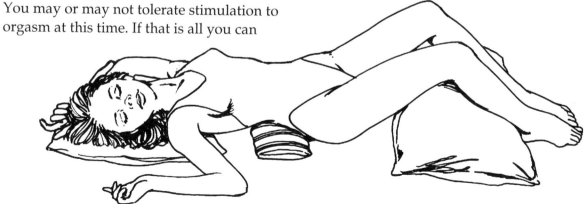

Figure 1

This back support pad may be moved about slightly during sex to achieve a variety of resting postures. Frequently shifting position, even slightly, can do a lot to minimize pain.

The back pain sufferer can maintain relaxation in this position while each partner shares a variety of sexual stimulation. This may be more comfortable than actual genital sex and can include a whole realm of touching, massage, oral sex, vibrator and other erotic play. Make this an opportunity to explore your sexuality and sensuality together.

The partner with the back problem may experience pains as the other partner moves about, shifting and tilting the mattress. You may wish to lie on a well-padded floor to avoid these upsets in the comfort of your lovemaking. Seemingly minor things like this can make the difference between pain or no pain. Make each unusual modification a part of the erotic atmosphere of your encounter.

Pain or the fear of pain can get in the way of pleasure and orgasm. You should proceed with sex with a great deal of patience and leisure. You should not be rushed and must avoid frustration. Gentleness should become an important part of your sex. Plan to take frequent breaks to change position or do some stretching and relaxation exercises to keep pain away.

Remember that the problem affects both of you. Try to help each other through the difficult moments. Keep your efforts relaxed and be patient with yourself and your partner. Let pain come and go without frustration. Avoid forcing yourself or your partner to perform too much. Talk. View all attempts as successful, despite their outcomes. Do not fear that your sexual future is doomed. Pay attention to what you can do together today and let this bring future success to your relationship.

Figure 2

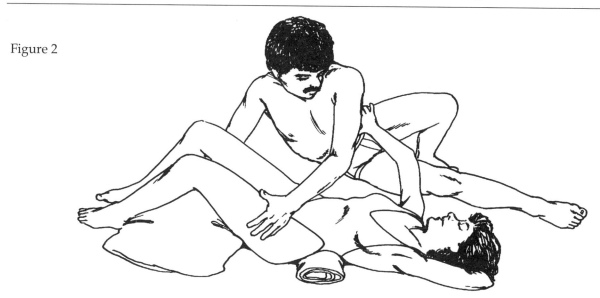

Actual genital intercourse may be too stressful to attempt at this stage until back pain is more under control. Sex during this very painful period may need to be limited to other forms of stimulation in the relaxed position described. Use this opportunity to explore your erotic alternatives. There are many ways to share gentle sexual love. Enjoy playing erotically with each other (Figure 2).

Cautious genital intercourse may eventually be attempted when you both feel ready. You should share lots of foreplay before such attempts. This will improve your enjoyment of sex while controlling back stress. Do not be in a rush to proceed beyond what your back can tolerate. Proceed only as you prove to yourself what you can handle without a setback. Proceed only as you both agree it is safe to proceed. Agree that encountering pain will not be met with anger or guilt by either of you, even if the pain brings this encounter to a halt.

57

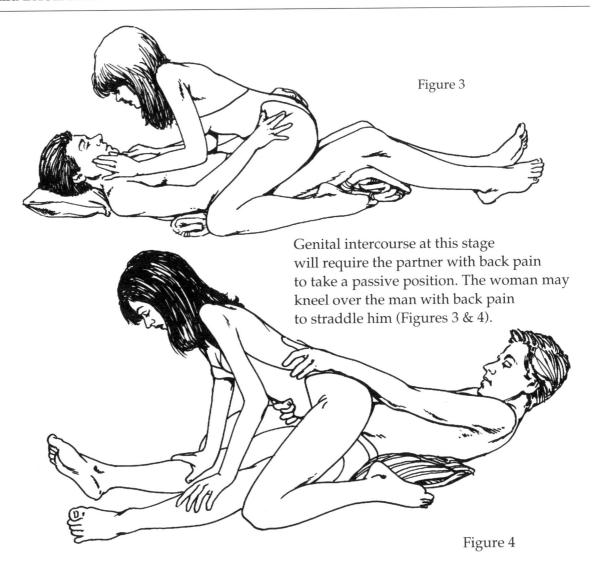

Figure 3

Genital intercourse at this stage
will require the partner with back pain
to take a passive position. The woman may
kneel over the man with back pain
to straddle him (Figures 3 & 4).

Figure 4

The man may approach the woman with back pain using the so-called "missionary" position as she maintains her legs comfortably bent (Figure 5). Be very gentle at this stage. The man or woman with the back problem should remain lying supine on his/her back as the partner mounts atop, as illustrated, for genital intercourse.

Oral sex and other stimulation also can be provided by the "passive" partner lying on his/her back with the partner on top assuming a variety of kneeling positions next to or over the back sufferer.

Figure 5

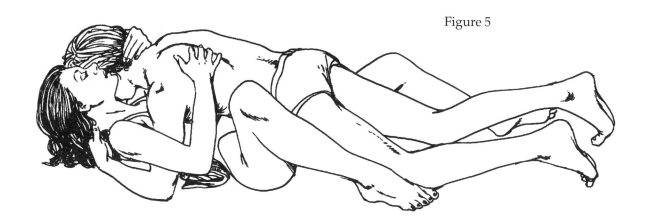

Figure 6

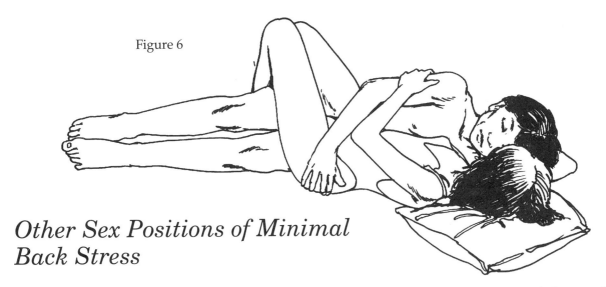

Other Sex Positions of Minimal Back Stress

Figure 6 is for either the man or the woman with back pain. The woman lies on her back while the man lies on his side beside her, facing toward her. She bends her legs up enough to allow him to bring his legs forward, underneath hers. She then rests her legs down over his. He can now enter her from this position. He can control the position of his back during intercourse by how he places himself next to her. She also has her back in a very relaxed position.

He may bend himself forward closer to her or lean back away from her to keep his back comfortable. She also can control the position of her back by how she positions her legs and by placing a small towel roll under her lower back. This allows them to proceed in as relaxed a manner as they wish. They are now in a good position for gentle sexual communication, face-to-face and easily able to touch one another.

Figure 7 is also for either the man or the woman with back pain. The woman lies on her side, back to him. The man lies on his side facing her back. The front of his body now rests against the back of her body as he approaches her from behind.

He can control the position of his back during intercourse by how he places his body next to hers. He may place himself close or away from her to control his position. She can control the position of her back by bending her body slightly forward to bring her chest down toward her knees, or by arching her back backward toward him. They are now in a relaxed position that allows touching and communication. She may rotate back slightly to face him, or may turn slightly toward her belly to further control position comfort.

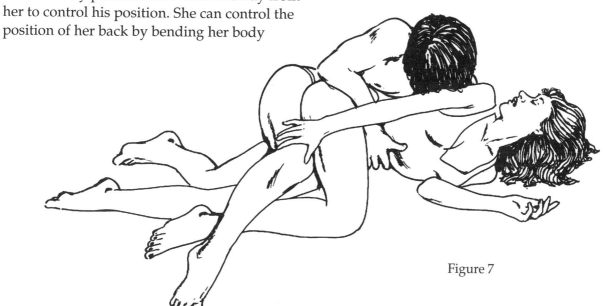

Figure 7

Summary

This "brittle" back pain stage can be frightening and frustrating. You hurt. You are afraid. You and your partner may be angry with

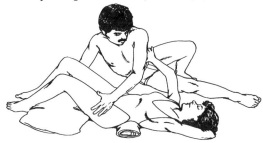

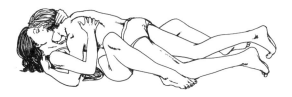

yourselves and each other. This can be a crisis stage. Your strategy for recovery of your sexual and loving relationship should be relaxed, open, planned and discussed between you.

Attention must be paid to developing effective pain control to be used before, during and after sex. This may even be incorporated into your sensual preparations and foreplay. Much

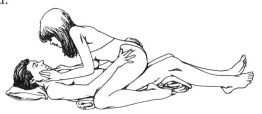

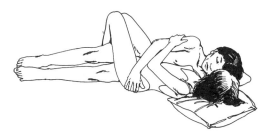

emphasis must be placed on foreplay stimulation. Erotic touch, massage, vibrators or oral sex may be the only sexual activity you can tolerate. Learn how to position yourselves to play with one another comfortably.

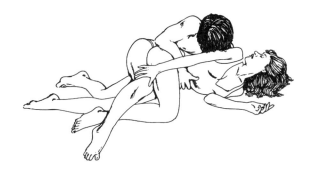

Several low-stress sex positions have been suggested. You should be able to gently and comfortably slip from one position to another and back again. Let foreplay stimulation bring you close enough to climax to minimize the physical demands of genital intercourse.

Sex Techniques for the Chronic Back Sufferer

You can use the Flexion Principle or the Extension Principle of back pain control to develop sex techniques for the man or woman with back pain.

People with chronic or recovering back conditions have varying degrees of ability and comfort. They also have various types of back problems. Some have chronic joint injuries that tolerate only certain movements and positions. Others have disc problems that tolerate different movements and positions. People with ligament sprains and muscle problems have their individual limitations. You need to understand how your spine works and how your specific back problems behave. You can use this knowledge to protect your back during various activities, including sex.

Every back problem behaves differently. Some back problems hurt more when the spine is bent *forward*, pulling and stressing certain

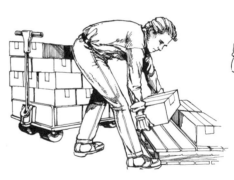

structures such as ligaments and discs. These problems usually feel better with the spine bent *backward* a little to relieve that stress. Other back problems, however, are made worse when the spine is bent *backward*, pinching and stressing other tissues such as joints.

These problems often feel better to have the spine bent *forward* a little to ease that stress.

A bulging or ruptured disc, for example, may be made worse when the spine is bent forward causing the disc to bulge more. Painful or arthritic joints often hurt more to have the spine bend backward, pinching the joints together. It is this pain behavior we will use to identify comfortable positions for sex.

Bending the spine forward (flexion) pulls on the muscles and ligaments while placing pressure on the disc. Strained muscles and ligaments may hurt more to be pulled in this manner. A bulging disc also may be damaged further by this position.

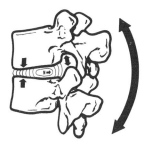

Bending backward (extension) eases the tension on the muscles and ligaments and reduces disc stress. Backward bending, how-

ever, causes the sensitive facet joints to pinch together. Joint problems, therefore, may hurt to be bent backward. Joint problems usually hurt less if the spine is bent forward at least slightly.

You can use this pain behavior to control your back stress. You can avoid movements and positions during sex that strain painful back structures. Back problems that hurt more during forward bending will do better when the spine is arched or bent somewhat backward, particularly during sex. Back problems that hurt with even slight backward bending generally feel better when the spine is bent forward. The sex positions we suggest use back postures that you can explore to maintain comfort during sex. That is the strategy of this book.

Physical therapists often classify back problems into two groups: **Flexion Principle** and **Extension Principle.** These are very broad classifications that do not fit everyone. Most back problems, however, fall into one of these two categories. Therefore, this classification system is useful to us in this book.

Flexion Principle simply means that the person hurts less to bend forward (flexion) and hurts more to bend backward. **Extension Principle** simply means it hurts less to bend backward (extension) and more to bend forward. We will classify sex positions into Flexion Principle or Extension Principle to identify sex techniques for women with back problems and again for men with back problems.

The back pain sufferer who fits the Flexion Principle will generally need to use sex positions that bend the lower back slightly forward. The normal inward arch of the lower back is actually flattened or bent out slightly in such a position.

People who fit the category of Extension Principle will need positions for sex that allow their lower backs to remain somewhat arched inward for slight backward bending. They usually have less pain when they keep their low back in its normal or slightly increased lordosis curvature.

Whether you will do better with positions that fit Flexion Principle or Extension Principle can only be estimated by your doctor or physical therapist. Only your cautious trial-and-error will tell you for sure which positions will work best for you. You can usually determine which category, Flexion or Extension Principle, best fits you by trying a simple test for discomfort in test positions used by physical therapists.

First, lie on your back. Carefully curl your knees toward your chest. Grasp and hold them toward your chest for up to ten seconds. Quit the position as soon as you encounter pain. Note your degree of discomfort.

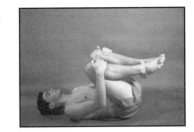

Now relax and gently turn over onto your belly. Cautiously prop up on your forearms to slightly arch your lower back backwards. Note your discomfort.

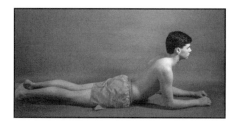

Repeat the test in the standing position. Standing upright, bend forward at the waist slowly and gently as far as is comfortable. Then resume upright posture.

Now bend backward gently, only as far as comfort allows. Note the difference in comfort between the two positions.

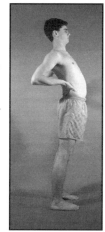

You fit **Flexion Principle** if curling your knees to your chest is more comfortable than lying on your belly propped up on the forearms, and if bending forward at the waist is more comfortable than bending backward while standing.

You fit **Extension Principle** if lying on your belly propped up on forearms is more comfortable, and if bending mildly backward while standing is more comfortable than bending forward.

If all these movements produce pain, you have a very stiff and sensitive spine that needs to reduce pain sensitivity, develop relaxation and restore flexibility. You probably will need to stick with the previously-described strategies for the "brittle" back until you restore more flexibility. You likely need professional therapy advice to help you rehabilitate your back.

The sex techniques we will describe next are placed in the categories of Flexion Principle or Extension Principle, for the man or woman with back pain. Start with those positions recommended by your therapist, or those you

67

feel you can handle based on how your back pain behaves with forward-bending or backward-bending test positions. Proceed slowly and gently.

As you proceed with sex, your strategy should be to place emphasis on relaxation, sensuality and foreplay. The object is to build up to physical sex in ways that avoid painful stress on your back. Use stimulation and touch to preserve your back and increase your pleasure. Proceed in a relaxed, gentle manner and let confidence and care replace anxiety and fear of pain as you gradually build your sexual abilities. Progress through the described sexual methods in a deliberate manner. Agree to try not to get frustrated or angry when you encounter pain or difficulty. Work on this together.

Be aware that the sex positions we will describe for people who need Flexion or Extension Principle will not be consistently successful. People often do not fit neatly into such categories. You will find some of our suggestions will work well, while others do not. You also may discover that your back pain does not

behave consistently on a day-to-day basis. What works today may not work tomorrow. We will later describe sex positions that do not fit either the Flexion or Extension Principles. These will be for people who need other special considerations.

You also will find that certain positions work well only if you do not sustain them for too long. Be willing to change positions often enough to avoid strain and fatigue. When you feel pain, try to determine if it was due to the wrong position or too much time in one position or was it simply fatigue?

Some people do not tolerate much movement. Other people do not tolerate holding still. Some do not tolerate lying on a tender back. Others do not tolerate lying on tender hips. Learn how your back pain responds to moving versus lying still, as well as specific positioning. Fit this pain behavior into your sexual strategies.

The Woman with Back Pain

*The woman with back pain can use the
Flexion Principle or Extension Principle
to discover positions for comfortable sex.*

This chapter describes sex positions for the woman with back pain. It is divided into two sections. One is for the woman who needs to keep her back slightly extended (Extension Principle). The other section is for the woman who needs to keep her back flexed forward for comfort (Flexion Principle). These are somewhat advanced techniques designed for those women who find they seem to fit either the Flexion Principle of Extension Principle of back pain behavior. Women with more severe pain or very unstable back problems may need to rely more on to the earlier chapter on "Sex Techniques for the Brittle Back".

Extension Principle Positions for Sex: (Women)

This describes sex positions for the woman who is more comfortable keeping her back supported in an arched or extension position. The objective is for her to preserve and support the arch in her lower back during sex.

A. The traditional missionary position described earlier (Figure 5) may not be comfortable for you unless your lower back is supported in an arched position. You can place a flattened towel roll or small pillow under your lower back for support. Your legs should not be bent up very far. Remember that you want to keep your lower back arched slightly. Experiment to determine which way is more comfortable for you before you begin.

Keep in mind that the firmness of a mattress you are using will affect the position of your back. A mattress that sags too much can strain the position of your back. A padded floor may be the more comfortable surface to try at first.

Do not be discouraged if you find that you cannot handle this traditional position for now. View it, instead, as an opportunity to explore new and different ways to experience and share pleasure. There are many positions and activities you can share that are not only less stressful to your back, but are also new and exciting.

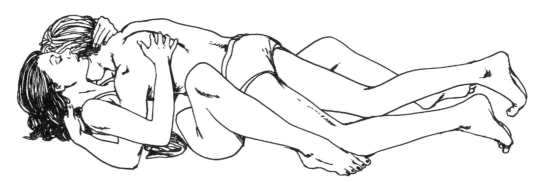

Figure 5

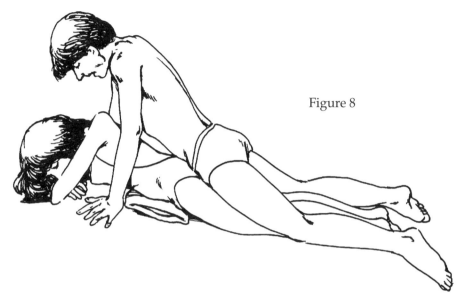

Figure 8

B. You may find it more comfortable to lie on your stomach and have your partner enter from behind (Figure 8). The simple act of lying on your belly places your back in a mild amount of extension. More extension can be achieved by placing a pillow at your chest or by propping up on your elbows. If you find you are more comfortable with slightly less extension, you can place a pillow under your stomach. You should try both of these modifications before lovemaking to discover which is most comfortable for you.

You may need to shift a pillow under you frequently during lovemaking to vary the position of your back and remain comfortable. By moving a pillow from beneath your chest to your belly and back again you will be able to have a variety of back postures that might reduce position discomfort.

Again, be aware that the firmness of a mattress will affect the position of your back. A mattress that sags too much can strain your back by extending it too far.

C. You may find sex to be more comfortable if you try sitting in your partner's lap while he sits in an armless chair. You may sit straddling him face to face (Figure 9) or with your back to him (Figure 10). You will be able to control your posture and movements in this position to find what is most comfortable for you. You may find it comfortable to either rock your pelvis or to move your entire body to create stimulation without actually moving your spine. This particular position offers the opportunity for a great deal of touching and sensual expression.

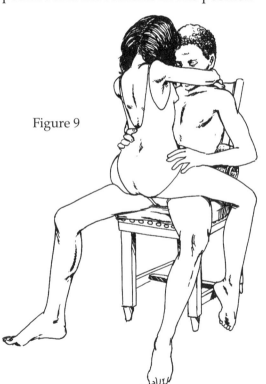

Figure 9

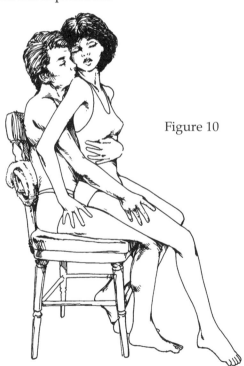

Figure 10

Be certain to select a chair of comfortable height and width. A low chair with a narrow seat will allow you to control your position by shifting your weight from your partner's lap to your feet. You may pad the seat to keep your partner more comfortable. It may be necessary to try several chairs to find one that is most comfortable for both of you.

D. There are several variations on the position discussed in Figure 8 that may allow you to actively adjust the posture of your lower back. You may find these variations helpful in controlling stress and discomfort.

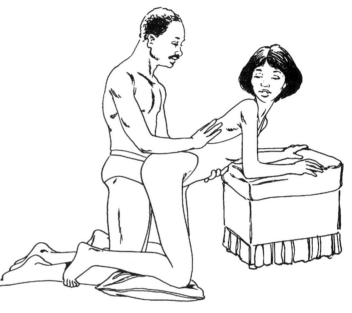

You can position yourself on your hands and knees on the bed or floor so that your partner can enter from behind. You also can kneel on the floor next to the bed or sofa and rest your upper body on your arms in a more upright posture. You will find that you can vary your back posture easily in either of these positions.

Be sure to cushion your and your partner's knees with pillows in this position. Not only will you be more comfortable, but these pillows also can adjust your heights to help you fit together better.

Figure 12

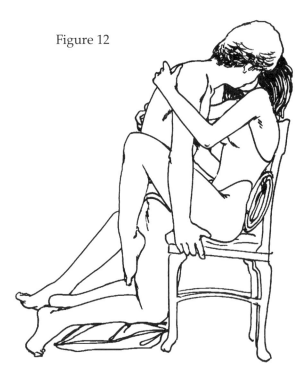

E. You may find it particularly relaxing and comfortable to enjoy making love in a semi-reclining sitting position (Figure 12).

Try sitting on a chair or sofa and slide your hips to the edge. You may place one or more pillows at your back so that you can recline backward, supporting your lower back. Ex-periment to discover how to place these pillows to provide you with the most comfort. Your partner can kneel between your legs for stimulation or intercourse. You can rest your feet on the floor or raise your knees toward your chest to control your comfort and vary your back position.

F. You can use the Extension Principle to position yourself for mutual manual or oral foreplay. Lie on your back with a folded pad under your lower back to support your lumbar arch (Figure 2). Your partner can then kneel over you to give or receive stimulation.

You also may kneel over your partner while he lies on his back, but remember to keep your back arched somewhat inward. You will then be able to maintain control of your back posture while you share a variety of stimulation (manual, oral, vibrator, etc.).

These positions, with one of you kneeling over the other, will allow you to change positions frequently to maintain comfort, as well as switch from passive to active roles in giving and receiving pleasure.

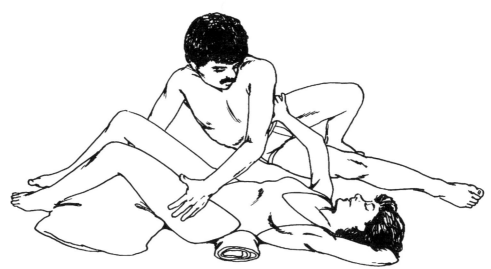

Figure 2

Flexion Principle Positions for Sex: (Women)

This section describes positions for the woman who finds comfort in keeping her back bent *forward*. How you position your legs can help position your back. Bending your legs up tends to bend your lower back forward. Keeping your legs straight tends to straighten your lower back.

A. The traditional missionary position is a flexion principle position for women. When you are lying on your back with your legs bent you will be able to maintain considerable flexion of your spine. You will find that you can control the amount of flexion by how far you bend your legs up toward your chest (Figure 5).

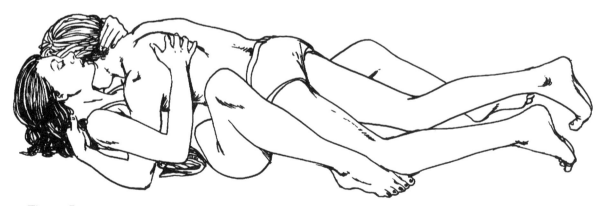

Figure 5

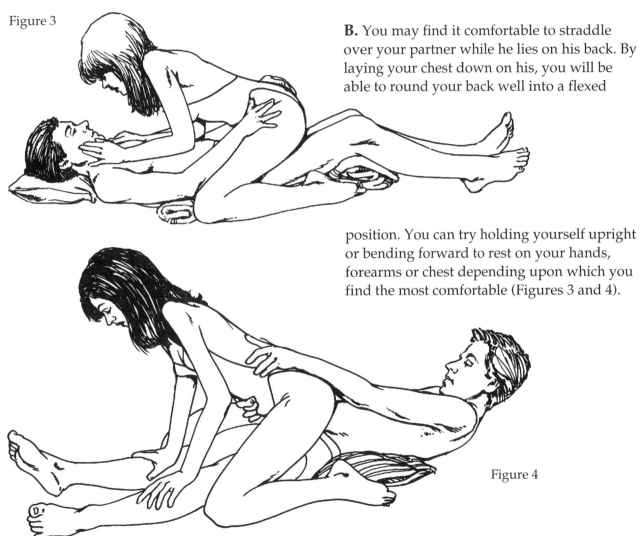

Figure 3

B. You may find it comfortable to straddle over your partner while he lies on his back. By laying your chest down on his, you will be able to round your back well into a flexed position. You can try holding yourself upright or bending forward to rest on your hands, forearms or chest depending upon which you find the most comfortable (Figures 3 and 4).

Figure 4

77

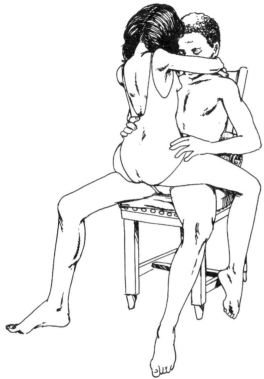

chair should be low enough to allow you to control how much weight you rest on your partner's lap versus on your feet on the floor. This will offer you control over your back stress.

These positions are similar to that described in the Extension Principle section with one important difference. Using the Flexion Principle you want to position yourself so that your back is bowed outward rather than arched inward. These positions offer you considerable control over your posture, whichever principle you are using, simply by consciously keeping your back rounded forward or arched inward.

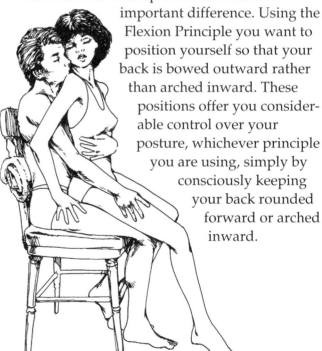

C. If you find you are comfortable with a Flexion Principle position, you may want to try sitting on your partner's lap while he sits in a sturdy chair. Try sitting both facing him and with your back to him to determine which position offers you the most control of your spine. Curl your spine or pelvis into whatever position seems most comfortable for you. The

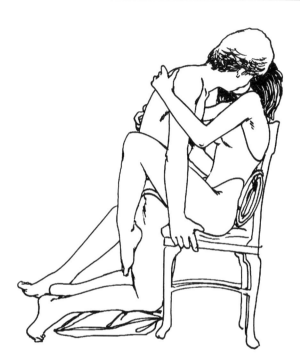

D. As described in the previous section, you may find stimulation or intercourse in a semi-reclining position comfortable and relaxing. The key is in controlling the position of your spine by how you prop your back with supportive pillows.

Try sitting on a chair or sofa with your hips placed all the way forward to the edge. In the flexion position you will want to use less or even no pillows behind your back. Remember, you want your back to be bent outward rather than inward for Flexion Principle positioning. You can control just how much your back is bent by the placement of pillows and by how you position your legs.

79

E. You may position yourself for stimulation or oral sex in the flexion position by lying on your back on the bed or floor with a pillow under your head and one under your knees. Keep your legs curled up comfortably. You may want to try this position at first with no padding under your lower back. The more comfortable you are, the more relaxed you will be.

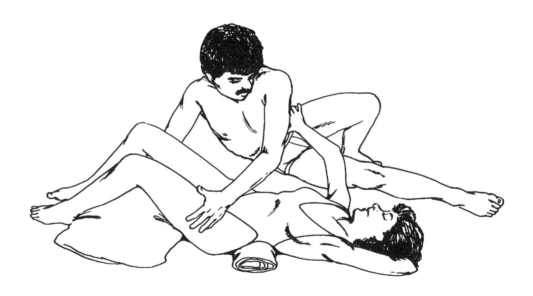

The Man with Back Pain

The man with back pain can use
the Flexion Principle and Extension Principle to
find positions in which he can comfortably enjoy sex.

This chapter describes positions that may help the man with back pain find comfort during sex. This is divided into a section on Extension Principle for men who find comfort keeping their back extended or arched, and a section on Flexion Principle for men who find comfort in bending the spine slightly flexed or rounded forward. These are rather advanced techniques. The man with severe or unstable back pain may need to start with techniques described in the earlier chapter, "Sex Techniques for the Brittle Back".

Extension Principle Positions for Sex: (Men)

This section describes sex positions that allow the man with back pain to keep his lower back arched, or extended backward slightly.

A. The traditional missionary position may or may not be comfortable for you depending upon the firmness of the mattress, your partner's position, how you support your body and how you both change positions. You may need to support yourself on your hands so that your lower back is arched *inward* somewhat. This may become tiring to your arms after a while, requiring good endurance and changes in positioning.

Your partner can help you by bending her legs toward her chest or placing a pillow under her buttocks so her pelvis is tilted up toward you. Whether you are comfortable in this position or not depends upon how you "fit" together during sex. The firmness of the bed also will affect your back position and comfort. You will want to experiment gently in this position at first.

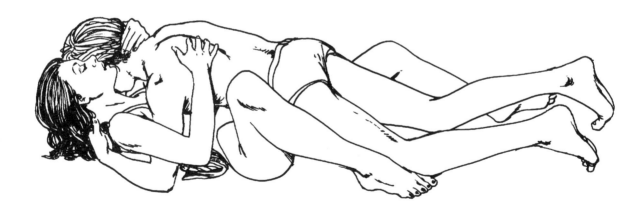

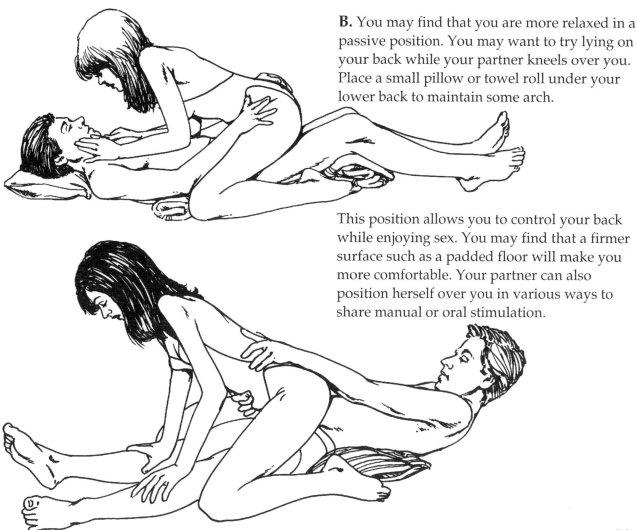

B. You may find that you are more relaxed in a passive position. You may want to try lying on your back while your partner kneels over you. Place a small pillow or towel roll under your lower back to maintain some arch.

This position allows you to control your back while enjoying sex. You may find that a firmer surface such as a padded floor will make you more comfortable. Your partner can also position herself over you in various ways to share manual or oral stimulation.

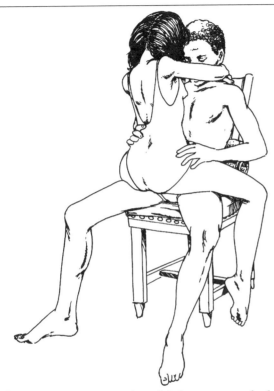

Many people with back problems find that they cannot sit for long periods of time. You should be prepared to change positions if you begin to notice any discomfort. A pillow beneath your buttocks will provide padding and allow a degree of ease in shifting position. You may need to try several different chairs to find one that is best suited for this position.

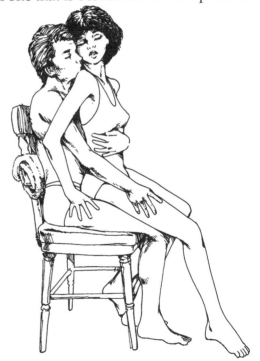

C. Another position in which you may feel comfortable is sitting on a sturdy chair with your partner on your lap straddling you. She can sit facing you or with her back toward you, depending upon which position the two of you find more comfortable. Place a small pillow or towel roll behind your lower back to maintain the normal arch.

84

Flexion Principle Positions for Sex: (Men)

This describes sex positions that keep your lower back rounded or bent slightly forward.

A. If you need to use the Flexion Principle you may find that the traditional missionary position is not comfortable for you if it arches your back too much. There are modifications that can help make this position more comfortable for you. Have your partner lie on her back with her legs bent. You may want to place one or two pillows beneath her back and buttocks. The pillows will raise her up enough for you to be able to draw up your knees and kneel between her legs (Figure 13). She can have her legs fully flexed or leave them down depending upon which gives you both the better "fit". You can enter your partner from this crouched position.

People are all built differently and you will need to experiment to find the "fit" that is most comfortable for both of you. It may be somewhat difficult to maintain this position for a prolonged period of time since reduced circulation in your legs may force you to change position. Plan to switch your positions as frequently as necessary to preserve your comfort.

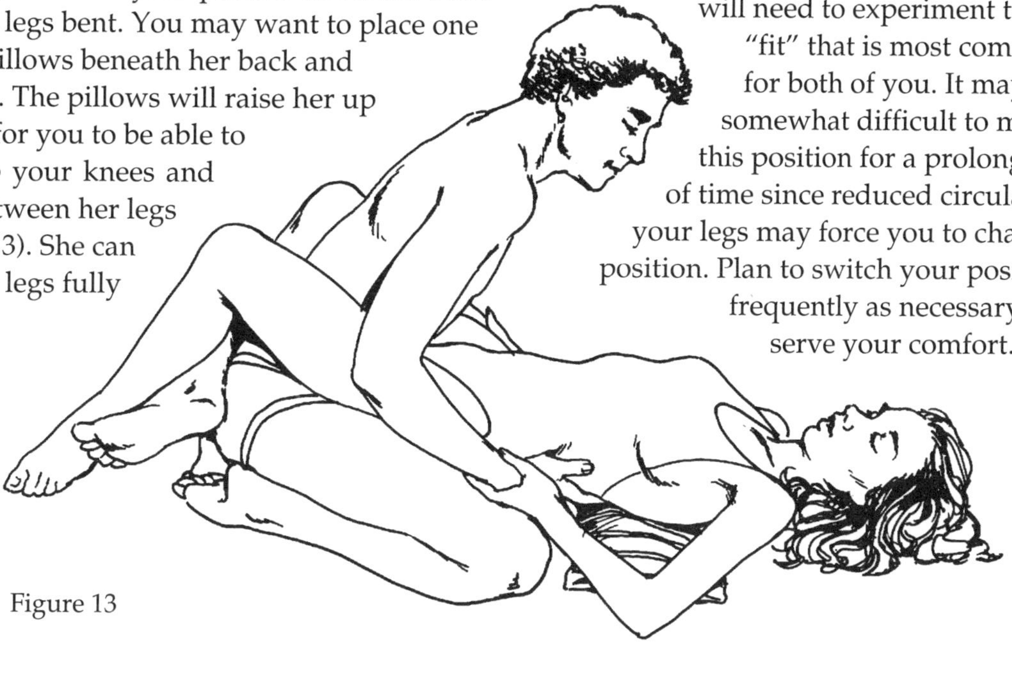

Figure 13

85

B. You may discover that you have greater control over the position of your back if you and your partner both kneel and you enter from behind. This will allow you to keep your back rounded out.

In this position you both kneel on a bed or on the floor. Kneeling on the floor as your partner props herself up on the side of the bed will create a variety of positioning possibilities as well as balance support for you both. Use pillows to cushion your knees on the floor and to make corrective adjustments in your height differences.

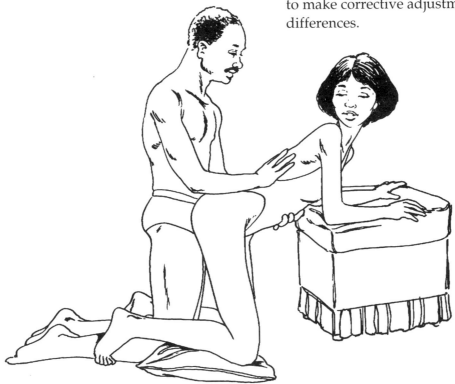

C. You will be able to give or receive various forms of sexual stimulation by kneeling over your partner while she lies on her back or by having her kneel over you in the same manner. If you lie on your back, either on the bed or floor, you will want to keep your legs slightly bent so that your spine will be flexed.

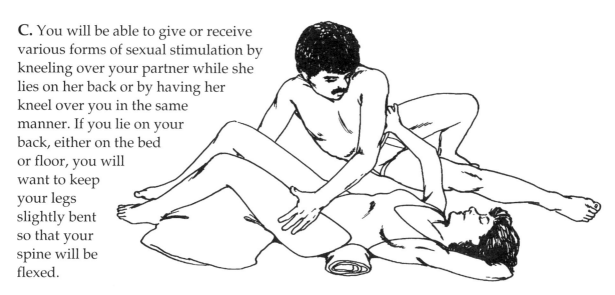

In this position you will be able to enjoy various forms of stimulation before actual intercourse, which will save your back's endurance.

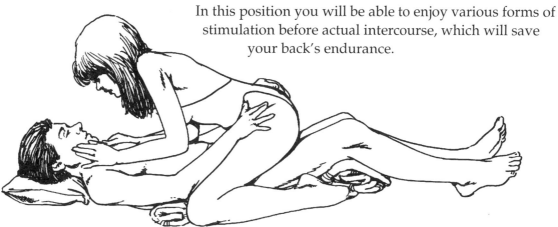

Other Positions and Methods

Not all back problems will fit Flexion Principle or Extension Principle. This is especially true of sacro-iliac, hip and other one-sided problems. These usually call for sex positions with one leg flexed and the other leg extended.

The previous chapters describe positions that fit into categories of Extension Principle or Flexion Principle of back positioning. Many back pain sufferers, however, do not fit either of these categories. They need other approaches to finding comfortable sex.

This chapter describes sex positions that do not specifically emphasize flexion or extension. These may meet the needs of back pain sufferers who do not fit the Flexion or Extension Principles. Furthermore, people who **do** fit Flexion or Extension categories also may benefit from these alternative techniques.

Many people have back problems affecting only one side of their spine. These include sprains or other arthritic problems of the facet joints or sacro-iliac joints. The facet joints connect the vertebrae to one another. The sacro-iliac joints connect the spine to the pelvis and hips. These joints are in pairs, located on each side of the spine. People with problems affecting these structures typically have pain on one side of the low back, often down into one hip.

The techniques to be described next are for people with pain affecting one side of their back, particularly involving a sacro-iliac sprain. This usually calls for the back pain sufferer to position himself/herself so that the leg on the painful side is bent up. The leg on

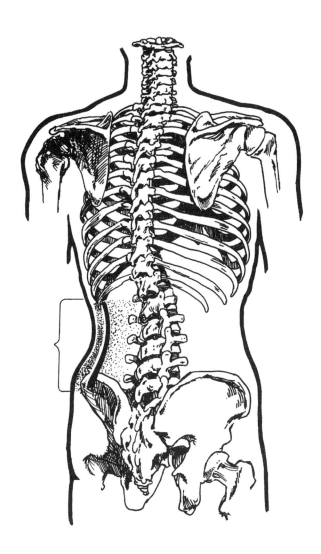

the pain-free side is kept flat or straight. This, of course, does not consistently fit everyone but it is a good starting point for your own exploration. A few people find that just the opposite position is better (pain-free leg bent up with pain-side leg out straight).

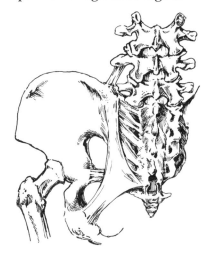

You should check out this approach with a simple test of positioning for comfort for yourself. Simply lie on your back and bend one knee up toward your chest (preferably the knee from the same side as your back pain). Hold this knee against your chest for ten to fifteen seconds as you judge this position to be comfortable or not. Then switch to holding your other knee to your chest with the pain-side leg down flat to decide which is more

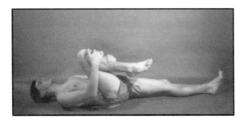

comfortable. Apply your pain behavior to the sex positions to be suggested next, keeping one knee flexed and the other straight to fit your comfort needs.

Any sex position will become painful if it is forced or prolonged. As lovemaking proceeds in a comfortable position, be willing to move to alternative positions to prevent discomfort. Learn when to switch positions before pain interrupts lovemaking.

Sex Positions for Men and Women with One-Sided Joint Problems

A. Any position in which you both lie on your sides will usually cause the least amount of back stress for both of you. The woman should lie on her back while he lies on his side next to her and facing her. She can bend up her leg closest to him so that he can bend his top leg forward and place it under her bent leg. She can then lay her leg down to rest atop his. Each partner should have one leg bent and one leg straight as he enters her from this position (Figure 14). You will want to experiment to determine which side you should lie on for maximum comfort. You will find that this is a comfortable and relaxed position that creates a pleasurable atmosphere for touching and communication. Use this opportunity to help each other relax and feel stimulated.

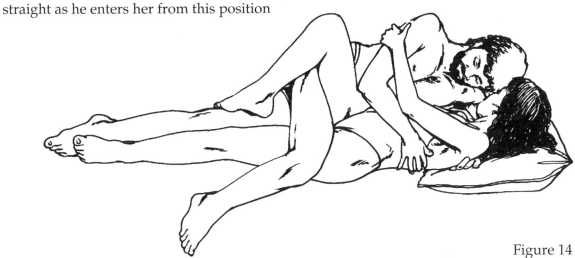

Figure 14

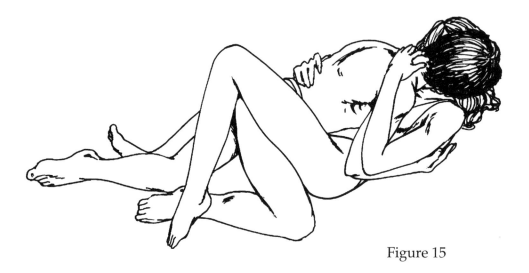

Figure 15

B. The **woman** with a one-sided joint problem will need to modify the missionary position to accommodate her condition. You will find it considerably more comfortable if you lie on your back with one leg bent up and the other leg lying flat (Figure 15).

C. The **man** with this problem also can modify the missionary position to suit his needs. Place yourself between her legs with one leg fully flexed and the other leg kept straight behind you (Figure 15). Place a pillow beneath your partner's buttocks if you find it more comfortable with her pelvis raised.

D. The **woman** with a one-sided back problem can also modify the semi-reclining, sitting position to enjoy more comfortable sex. Try sitting on a sofa or easy chair with your buttocks positioned up to the edge. Bend one leg up and place the heel of that foot on the edge of the seat while keeping your other leg down and your foot on the floor. Your partner can then kneel between your legs. You may place a pillow behind your back to keep it stable and in the most comfortable position.

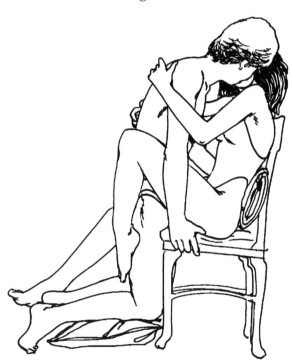

Sexual Apathy

Back pain and its effects can lead to sexual apathy.
This is part of the challenge of your recovery!

It is not unusual for a back problem to create a kind of sexual apathy. You are in pain, depressed and insecure, often suffering from low self-esteem. This negative state of mind can occasionally result in a reduced interest in sexual activity or even a total loss of desire. You may feel confused and guilty about this and your partner may feel the same. He or she may feel that they are somehow responsible for your lack of sexual desire. This can be a difficult and potentially painful situation for both of you.

There are many possible reasons for this kind of sexual apathy in either partner. Pain and/or fear of pain are often the primary causes of reduced sexual desire. Constant pain can often dominate your life, altering normal behavior and invading every aspect of your existence. You may never feel completely relaxed dealing

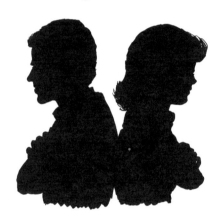

with your injury or pain in situations that you would normally find quite comfortable.

As the partner of the back pain sufferer, you may fear that you will cause your partner more pain during love making. Your partner's pain is mysterious to you; something you cannot truly share. You may feel unable to relax during sexual activity because you cannot stop worrying about the pain you may cause. These thoughts can be frightening and cause you to lose interest in trying at all.

You both must accept the presence of pain and take the necessary steps to minimize or eliminate it. Follow the steps for pain control and relaxation outlined earlier. Most importantly, communicate your doubts and fears to your partner. If you are experiencing pain, tell your partner and work together to deal with it. If you worry about inflicting pain, share that concern. Don't allow each other to remain in the dark and assume that each of you understands the other. This can lead to wrong conclusions which damage your relationship.

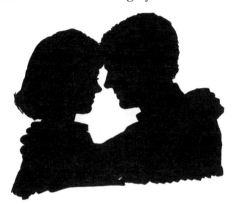

Sexual Apathy and Loss of Self-Esteem

Loss of self-esteem can be a major factor in sexual apathy. Perhaps your injury has restricted your activities to the extent that you sometimes feel useless and a burden to your family. You may be experiencing a great deal of guilt and anger with yourself because you are not working or cannot care for your family as you once did. It is difficult to feel good about your sex life if you don't feel good about yourself. You may feel that you have changed and are no longer desirable.

As the partner of someone with back pain you also may experience negative feelings directed toward yourself. You feel guilty because your loved one is suffering and you are unable to help. You may even feel responsible in some

95

way because your partner is injured. You may feel that your sexual desire for your partner is selfish and uncaring. When your loved one is angry at their pain, you may imagine that he/she is angry with you.

Loss of self-esteem can severely cripple an otherwise healthy, loving relationship. The kinds of negative feelings that result from low self-esteem can often be quite difficult to share with your partner. But talking about your feelings is always better than letting your partner try to guess what you are feeling. Low self-esteem can cause loss of the motivation necessary for a speedy and full recovery. A negative view of yourself can lead to a negative view of your condition and a feeling of hopelessness. This is a situation that will endanger your recovery and your relationship with your family. If either or both of you are experiencing a loss of self-esteem you must share those feelings and help each other to deal with them. You may find that you can help each other the most when you are feeling the most helpless. Remember that you are suffering with pain but are not responsible for

it. You need to share your doubts and dedicate yourselves to eliminating them together.

Sexual apathy can be dealt with if you invest the time and patience and have a genuine desire to share a full and meaningful sex life with your partner. If you had a satisfying sexual relationship before your injury, you can have one again.

If, however, you and your partner were experiencing difficulties within your relationship before your injury, the situation is likely to continue to deteriorate after your injury. You must distinguish sexual problems that are a result of your disability from relationship issues that existed before it. Has back pain become a convenient means of avoiding sex with your partner? Do not be afraid or ashamed to seek professional counseling. You may find that you can use this opportunity to rebuild your relationship with your partner and make it better than it was before.

Sexual Apathy in Men with Back Pain

The man who is suffering from back pain may feel physically helpless. You may feel that you have become a useless burden if you are accustomed to taking care of your family and those responsibilities requiring physical strength. Your sense of self and your ego can be severely damaged by your physical injury.

It is important to understand the difference between apathy and impotence, which will be discussed later. Apathy is a lack of interest in sexual activity, not an inability to perform. Apathy may be caused by a fear of failure or a general lack of self-esteem. You may feel that in loosing some of your physical abilities you have also lost your appeal for your partner. You feel that you are less than what you once were.

You must try to remember that your pain is not you. Don't define yourself by your disability. Concentrate instead on the process of regaining what you have lost. Be patient with yourself. Give yourself a chance. Don't be afraid to talk with your partner about your doubts. Dedicate yourself to returning normalcy to your life step by step. You may find that you are strong in ways that you did not realize.

Impotence

A back problem may occasionally present complications that can lead to episodes of impotence. Impotence has been traditionally labeled as every man's greatest fear. Loss of ability to achieve or maintain an erection can strike any man at any time with or without the complications of a painful injury. Impotence can be a complication of back pain and should not be viewed with panic, blame or guilt by either partner.

Pain or fear of pain can readily produce temporary impotence. A man who is afraid of causing his lover pain may be unable to per-

97

form sexually. Some medications used to treat back pain also may contribute to impotence. A few men with serious back problems may have nerve irritation or damage that can cause impotence.

Men who are out of work or physically restricted by back pain may develop feelings of inadequacy or worthlessness due to their disability. This can affect their ability to achieve an erection and even reduce their interest in sex. Inability to perform sexually can create increased anxiety and stress that in turn can create more pain and discomfort. Impotence is an area of human performance in which the mind and body greatly affect one another.

It is important that neither partner blame themselves or each other for these types of difficulties. Guilt and blame can make the situation worse! Impotence is usually another pain issue that will pass with the proper care and time. Give yourself the chance to recover fully and don't let impotence stop you from enjoying successful sex play.

One strategy is to proceed with sexual activity without an erection. The penis is not a man's only sex organ! Oral sex, manual stimulation, vibrators and an emphasis on other sensual and erotic sex-play offer many alternatives worth exploring. Exploration of other methods of sexual expression could lead to many exciting new discoveries. This may be yet another opportunity disguised as a problem.

Sexual Apathy in Women with Back Pain

Just as men and women often have uniquely different ways of viewing their sexuality, they also can have different ways of viewing and dealing with pain.

As a woman you may not view your disability in terms of a loss of physical strength. Caring for your family can be a major part of your life whether or not you work outside the home.

You may feel a great deal of guilt and worth-lessness if you are not able to care for them as you once did. You may be unable to take the same kind of care of yourself to which you are accustomed and feel unattractive as a result. Perhaps you feel that you will be unable to satisfy your partner sexually and, therefore, unwilling to try. You may fear that your physical discomfort will cause your partner to find you unappealing. You may worry that he is too afraid of hurting you to find pleasure in your love-making. Perhaps your own fear of pain inhibits your desire to even attempt making love. All these factors can lead to sexual apathy and contribute to conflict.

Relaxation and focus is a vital part of a woman's satisfying sexual experience. You must be able to concentrate fully on that experience without the distraction of doubt or fear of pain. Accept that the pain exists and take the steps necessary to reduce or eliminate it. Let your partner help you in this. Tell your partner what is most comfortable and stimu-lating for you and when you need to stop to rest or deal with the pain. Don't be afraid to express your needs. This often adds more closeness to your love-making. View the process of recovery as a shared experience, including the recovery of your sex life.

Relaxation is often the key to achieving sexual arousal for a woman. Concentrate on the experience itself, rather than the factors that might detract from it. Accept the reality of the possibility of pain without anticipating it. Plan with your partner ahead of time how you will deal with it should it occur. Don't assume that your present sexual apathy means that you cannot be aroused. Focus on what makes you feel good. Don't be afraid to ask for patience or express your needs. Make this part of your sensuality.

Making It All Work

- *Communicate.*
- *Plan your strategy.*
- *Incorporate pain control into your sex activity.*
- *Expect success.*

Your back problem has placed itself in the way of your sex life. You can use relaxed attitudes, more open communications and new approaches to enjoying sex not only to recover what you have lost, but also to build a better sex life than you had before your back problem! Keep reminding yourself that every problem is an opportunity. You may discover something valuable that you otherwise would have missed. The relationship you recover may be even better than the one you had before your injury.

You will need to place an increased emphasis on foreplay, oral sex and other forms of erotic stimulation to save stress on your back. This will increase your sexual capabilities, options and tolerances. You also should place an increased emphasis on the sensuality and romance around lovemaking. The idea is to express your sensuality and sexuality with more than just genital intercourse. This helps you enjoy yourself and each other by reducing your attention to physical limitations and pain.

Just as with back exercises, you should proceed slowly at first and gradually build according to your comfort. Avoid sustaining any position or repeating any movement for a prolonged period of time. Proceed gently, planning to shift positions and techniques often. This is the best method of protecting your back during sex.

100

You may find it helpful to soothe and relax your back before attempting the physical demands of sex. Use whatever safe pain control methods you have available just before sexual activity. These include moist heat, ice, massage, stretching or relaxation exercises. Repeat these after sex to reverse any pain or discomfort encountered during sex. You may need to plan pain-control breaks during sex to enjoy the activity fully and safely.

When You Encounter Pain

You will need to agree ahead of time how you will respond when you encounter pain. Plan to stop at the first signs of fatigue and discomfort so that you may rest, relax and compose yourself. You may then be able to proceed. Agree up front that anger and frustration will not destroy the experience should pain bring love-making to a halt.

When you encounter pain, let the pain and your initial reactions subside. Then proceed with gentle massage, heating pad, ice massage, gentle stretching and relaxation exercises to share in bringing the pain under control. Try to do this together. Do not isolate one another. Accept that some anger and frustration may arise, but try to accept each small step forward as a kind of success. Rejoice in the attempt rather than despairing at failure. View each encounter as a positive step forward. You may be able to resume some gentle sexual activity after a few minutes of recovery. Just being able to move beyond any encounters with pain is substantial progress.

Working Together for Success

Remember that this problem and its resolution involves both of you. You must both decide to find solutions together. This must be a shared effort. Discuss it openly with one another. Take turns reading this book, perhaps underlining key statements and ideas that are important to point out to one another.

Agree that you will each devote an honest effort to make this successful. Agree to succeed. This is vital. Agree also that encountering difficulty or pain during any attempt to make love will not be viewed as a setback. Every time you express physical love you are making love, whether it works out exactly as you planned or not!

Rejoice in your attempts to make love and forget about any encounters with pain that forced you to stop. Do not allow blame or guilt or anger to come between you. Do not blame yourself or your partner. If anger or blame or guilt comes out, let it pass, let it go. Let it be a part of your back problem that will fade away as you proceed forward to rebuilding your life. Be patient with one another. Accept that anger and frustration may come and go. Communicate about it.

Plan to Succeed!

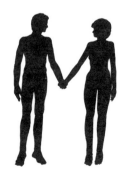